Develop The Mental Strength Of A Warrior For Success In Life

Gaurav Sanjiv Kalangan

Published by Gaurav Sanjiv Kalangan, 2024.

Also by Gaurav Sanjiv Kalangan

Learn Options Strategies Options Basics & Greeks For Stock Trading By Technical Analysis

Bitcoin, Altcoins & ICOs Learn the Basics of Digital Coins from Zero

Time Management This Is How I Work 300 Percent Faster

How To Build And Implement A Winning Pricing Strategy

Networking For Introverts: Gracefully Exiting A Conversation

Accounting 101: Learn Cost Accounting From A To Z

Growth Marketing: Strategy & Execution Bootcamp For Startups

Develop The Mental Strength Of A Warrior For Success In Life

Table of Contents

Copyright

Copyright© 2024 by BHARAT NISHAD.

Published by BHARAT NISHAD

Develop The Mental Strength Of A Warrior For Success In Life

Cover Design: BHARAT NISHAD

Cover Photo/illustration: BHARAT NISHAD

Layout & Design: BHARAT NISHAD

The accounts in this book are true and accurate to the best of our knowledge. They may contain some speculation by the author(s) and opinions/analyses from psychology, criminology, and forensics experts. This book is offered without guarantee on the part of the editor, authors, or publisher. The editor, authors, and publisher disclaim all liability in connection with the use of this book.

About

FEAR is one of the most elemental factors that can either make or break your own success. It can both stop you dead in your tracks and deprive you of your dreams, or you can push through fear to discover the true wealth of success on the other side of it.

When you look objectively at fear, you'll quickly notice that it only exists in your mind. It's only a thought. You can't hold fear in your hand. You can't pick it up off the ground. It's completely invisible and ONLY based on your own thinking and belief systems. Nothing more.

Everyone has unique fears embedded in their own subconscious minds, including yourself. These fears can suck the vitality and happiness out of your life in a hurry. It can also render you paralyzed when trying to push forward to achieve things you desire.

Fortunately, since fear is only based on your thinking and beliefs, with the right tools, techniques and guidance...you can defeat your fears once and for all.

Once you know how to become the MASTER of your fears, not only will you gain amazing control over your subconscious mind (which actually dictates your entire life)...but it'll also allow you to Develop the Mental Strength of a Warrior to get everything you want out of life.

The truth is, every solution to every problem or fear you have in life all begins WITHIN you, not outside of you. The golden keys that will unlock all the success and achievements you'll ever want in life are right there tucked away within yourself.

And the good news is, once you tap into your own powers to obliterate your fears, and gain the mental toughness and strength of a true warrior, your life will TRANSFORM.

Meet The Instructor and Goals

Hi buddy. This Book was designed to help people out who are having challenges in life which is virtually everybody, everybody has old hurts old pain. This Book is designed to give you freedom from pain to give you a joyous life, a life second to none. That's my wish for you. And today we're gonna teach you dozens and dozens of skills to make that a reality for you so you can have the life, the joy, the experience that you want to have and that you so richly deserve SO WON'T YOU PLEASE GIVE A WARM WELCOME.

Again, as you can tell from the background, I'd like to read a book or two on why I want to bring you cutting edge tools, strategies and techniques that can make a measurable and noticeable difference in the quality of your life both personally and professionally. I want to help you on every level. To do that I've constantly gotta be learning so I can constantly keep teaching and give you the highest quality skills available. Now here's just a few things that you're about to discover. One discovers how to understand and destroy old pain. We want to get rid of that old hurt that old pain for you.

Cut it completely out of your life. To build new and empowering beliefs and values to take you further than you ever thought possible. 3 eliminate old lies and misperceptions that are holding you back for game powerful new skills to help you excel in life. 5. Improve your relationship with both yourself and others. 6 learn how to control your mind in your emotions. How amazing would that be? How powerful would that be? 7 discover powerful secrets of psychology that have been hidden from you. You will know more about psychology after this Book than probably 99 percent of the country. 8 We want you to gain new freedom. We want you to love your life. Life is meant to be lived.

It's meant to be experienced. It's meant to be enjoyed not suffered through and number 9 I simply stayed here and so much more. Why? We've got dozens and dozens of very powerful, very targeted tools here for you. I couldn't begin to describe them in a single sheet in a single chapter and just a few minutes but you're gonna get this warm, deep , rich experience of going through each tool. Step by step in literally transforming your life. So a little bit about me. Who am I and how can I help? I've been on a mission for the last 35 plus years to help people like you excel both personally and professionally. That's why I do these chapter chapters.

Teaching is my joy. I want you to have advantages that I didn't have at your age. And most people go from the cradle to the grave from the womb to the tomb and never have these tools. So I want to make sure that I'm out there, that I'm sharing these with you and that you can have that beautiful life. We've been talking about it as a personal favorite of mine. Please share these skills with other people. Let them know about this Book and just teach them some of these things yourself to whom much is given much is expected when you get something that's really great in your life. You should share it with as many people as you can. Now just quickly, just a little bit about me and my background. You can always pause the chapter and read through it if you want but basically I'm a pretty smart guy.

I've got four different degrees in business and psychology. I'm the CEO of advanced ideas. I've been a corporate trainer for many many years. I also ran several multimillion dollar corporations largely in the healthcare field but some in business. I'm a trained psychotherapist. I was a licensed mental health counselor licensed drug and alcohol counselor in the state of New Hampshire. I'm a certified addiction professional in Florida so I've been doing therapy for many many years inpatient outpatient Intensive Outpatient partial hospitalization residential therapeutic communities Outward Bound anything you can think of. I pretty much have done it.

I'm a university professor. I've won multiple teaching awards and done that for many many years. I'm a six figure Internet marketer. I've read over 500 books. This doesn't even count the ones that I used to get the four degrees. So I read about four to five books every single month in psychology, business , health and all the major life areas so that I can bring you the best tools, the best strategies and the best techniques above and beyond that. I did another six thousand hours and probably up to seven or eight thousand hours now of additional chapters. So mentoring mastermind groups C.D. chapter any kind of information gathering that I could get to make sure that I become a stronger therapist, a stronger educator, stronger trainer again to bring you the cutting edge tool strategies techniques that are going to make an amazing difference in your life when you apply them.

Now I have the exact same goal that you do. My only goal is to help you grow to remove the barriers that have held you back and to teach you new cutting edge skills. If you follow and practice what I teach in this chapter you will excel now. My goal is to be a mentor to you. What is a mentor? Well one definition is a wise guy to make your path easier. It's kind of like I've been through the minefield and I can tell you where to step so you don't hit any of the landmines. There may be more ways to do it than that but if you follow my path you'll get through the other side. There's also an old phrase that says Let me have done that for you.

So any challenges that I've had in my life I'm going to show you how to get around those in your life. I'm also going to show you what's worked for people over and over and over again. I've had massive success rates with people in therapy and doing personal coaching to help them excel in life. So I can show you how to do this quickly and easily, taking years off your learning curve and saving a massive amount of pain, effort , money , finance and trouble. So my goal is to be a good mentor. A good mentor is a good friend. Here's another definition for you to write this down for your notes. My best friend is the one who brings out the best in me. That's my goal to bring out the best in you.

You've got excellence inside of you. It's only been covered up in just a couple of opening statements for ninety nine point seven percent of the people reading this chapter. Your depression, anxiety , low moods, low self-esteem whatever it may be for you. I want to tell you something and I want you to hear this clearly. It's not your fault. So in this chapter you'll learn what did cause it. And I'm going to show you the way out. Here's a great quote, another good one to put in your notes or go ahead and print out this screen. Nothing you achieve will ever be greater than what you are, what you were born as. Which is beautiful, innocent and perfect. You are born great. It has only been covered up. So the purpose of this chapter will be to uncover your greatness.

Release your natural state of happiness and serenity. Enjoy. I want you to have that life second in line to have a full deep rich experience of life. That's how it was supposed to be. We're going to get back to that. And you'll be amazingly happy in this amazing Book. You will learn so many fantastic skills. It will literally blow your mind. Now to make sure that that happens we need some concentration. So be sure to close any and all other windows, remove any distractions, cut down any noises and I want you to take excellent notes. People that mentally engage in it focus on it and take good notes. These people have three times the results.

So taking careful notes is important. Very important, it's going to triple your results. I want you to get the maximum out of this Book. This Book is designed to literally transform your life. You have nothing going on today that is more important than what you're going to learn inside this Book, quick little disclaimer for you. I want you to know this is not therapy. I'm not being hired on as your therapist. I'm simply giving you good solid advice. That's worked for me and my clients. Year after year after year bring you those cutting edge tools. If you need professional therapy please go out there and get it. I was a professional therapist like I said for decades. Find a good therapist that can help you if you need additional help.

This is not therapy. This is education. But education can be absolutely amazing and extremely powerful. But I want to make sure that nobody's left out they're floundering if they need more help in this Book, so I'm going to wrap this up here. This is just simply the intro and we are going to jump in. So I'm excited for you. You're going to learn some great strategies. Some things are going to make you feel absolutely fantastic. This is going to revolutionize your life. Again if you focus and if you apply it so you're doing fantastic I'm proud of you. And I'll see you in the very next chapter. We're going to jump in and we're going to learn skill after skill after skill all the way through the chapter. You will be amazed before you're halfway done. I'll see you there.

Beginning Concepts - Key Life Areas

Hey everybody welcome back breaking news don't live with problems solve them. When's a good time to solve them. Now they're going to say to me Hey I already know this actually and this will probably surprise you. You don't know this or maybe you know some people intimately that don't know this. Maybe you live with some people that don't know this. Think of it this way as a therapist. How do I know that you know something if you know something is a problem. Then you recognize it. You take massive action to solve it and then it's gone and you tell me about it later. Otherwise you don't know or your knowing does you no good.

But it's one of the others. So most people don't realize they have problems or if you bring it up they'll say Oh yeah I know that's a problem. No. When you know it you're motivated you're driven. Your brain will kick in and will solve virtually any problem that you know you have. It's part of your denial system that you have a problem and you say I know it. Air quotes are involved and you just relegate it to a back corner of your mind. We have to look at it again. So do you really know something that you've hidden from yourself?

The answer is no you don't really know it because if you knew it you would have jumped on it you know it you know it's important and you're not doing anything so you clearly don't quote unquote know it. You don't. The first step in getting rid of these problems is to accept that no you don't really know that you have a problem. Now step two is go ahead and solve them which means take massive action. Now for most people they can take massive action on their problems because they're so simple you're overweight. What you need to do. Eat less you smoke, get rid of everything that makes fire and stop smoking or switch to vaping. OK. And then drop down the nicotine levels and then get rid of it.

These are all simple solutions. You're in a bad relationship. Realize the door works and walk out of it. The problem is you're next to that person. Get the hell away from them. You're in a bad marriage. What's the solution? Go to therapy and solve it or get out. There's no third option except stay in it and be miserable when somebody says All I know I should leave No. If you knew you'd already be gone. You don't know you are relegated to the back of your mind. You don't take action, you don't solve it, which is the natural Book of things when you actually do know and recognize you have a problem, so problems are actually fairly simple to solve. My problem as a therapist is not figuring out how you're going to solve your problem, it's easy getting you motivated to take the actions to solve it.

That's wildly complicated. It takes a lot of motivational chapters and it takes a lot of effort on my part to motivate people to make the simple changes that they quote unquote now they need to make. So what are the methods that we use to make this habit? And what are the major life areas that we need to start dealing with. Let's take a look at some of the major life areas that we just really truly need to square away. These are the fundamentals the Prado principle says 20 percent of what you do creates 80 percent of your results. So this is the 20 percent of your life that creates 80 percent of your stress or 80 percent of your problems or we give you 80 percent of the benefits compared to taking care of 100 percent of everything. So these are the major life areas and they need to be addressed.

The first one is significant to others and this is in no particular order. Remember the quality of my life is the quality of my relationships. So to deal with significant others you need to make sure that you didn't make what's called a PPE. That's an old management term P P E point of purchase error you bought into the wrong person you got the wrong girl you've got the wrong guy it's never gonna work out why. Because you're not a therapist and you can't change them, they are never going to make it. They didn't have the right job qualifications and they're not willing to be retrained. You've gotta get rid of them, it's a PPE. Let me give you an analogy.

You have a spatula and all a sudden it breaks. So now you want to make yourself some pancakes or a tasty egg and you go down to Sears or you go down to Wal-Mart and you look for a spatula and you find some that kind of looks like a spatula. It's got a handle on it. It's got a long extension on it. It's got a flat head on it's called a screwdriver. You say Oh this is just like a spatula. Just a different style. I'll bring this home and it'll work. Then you get it home and you try to flip your pancake. You're trying to flip your egg with it; it just breaks it all up. What do you do? You don't try to retrain the screwdriver to be a spatula.

You don't try to go to a metal shop and you know an attachment to it or pound it into shape in a forge you know like your own games of thrones and do that type of thing. Here's what you do. Use another management term called sunk cost. You realize that this thing is never going to do the job. You grab the screwdriver you throw it in the trash you go back down to Wal-Mart you buy the correct tool you buy a spatula you come home and you have joy for the rest of your life you make yourself tasty pancakes and tasty eggs and everybody is very impressed with how they came out so well. Why?

Because you had the right tool. So with significant others, especially the person that's most important in your life, the man or the woman in your life, you've got to have the right person now assuming you have the right person. There may be issues. So get you some chapters, get you some self-help books or a lot of times you need to get into therapy. Therapy is just a legitimate shortcut. It makes it quicker and faster to do something that you may or may not have been able to do on your own. But even if you could do it on your own I'd rather have some of these issues solved in a month than me trying to do it over five or 10 years of my life. It just goes better in a therapy chapter situation. And the therapist can teach new skills that will not only solve the current problems you have but teach them more about life and solve future problems.

That's a great outcome. You have to deal with a significant other issue. There's an old expression I don't know where it comes from but it simply states if mama ain't happy ain't nobody happy. Which means you only got to have one negative significant other in your house in your life is going to be hell. You can have everything else going great, you can have money and looks and finances and a great career and be top of your field and when your significant other is unhappy they will make you miserable. You have to solve this major life area. A funny thing is a lot of people will come to me in therapy and they say I'm so anxious I'm so depressed I'm so miserable I can't seem to get ahead in life.

Nothing seems to be working for me. I just feel bad all the time. I have low self esteem and come to find out there's not a—thing wrong with them. It's their significant other you know whose spouse rhymes with louse that may not be an error. You know sometimes you just got a lousy spouse they got allowed isn't the way you pronounce it right. So they just need to get rid of that person or correct the issues that are going on in that relationship. Just remember that significant others are huge in your life. This is a problem that has to be solved. Now the jail is stumped , sometimes standing for just above broke just over broke right.

So jail is the job. This is where you spend the bulk of your time. You spent eight hours a day there. You got to take a shower before you went there . You got to drive there. It ends up being about 10 hours every single day. Even though you're only working 8 hours at least 5 days a week now some people can extend that another 10 or so hours to make it you know instead of 50 hours a week it's 60 or 70 or 80 hours a week. Some people even do stuff over the weekends so he gets very big very quickly. Now this becomes a huge part of your social life because you work on the job. So if you're being belittled on the job you don't feel good on the job. This is where you spend the bulk of your time. It can really damage you psychologically. And remember we said your purpose in life is very important.

A lot of people think their job is their purpose. That's not necessarily true. I'm in the helping field so my job can be my purpose in life but if I make toasters it's hard to turn that into my purpose in life. I can say well everybody needs toasters and toast just wouldn't get made in the world if it wasn't for me. Then I guess you can find a little satisfaction out of that but most people that are doing jobs that don't directly help somebody else in a really significant way. They find their purpose in life somewhere else. You know it has to do with their kids or it has to do with your charity work or mentoring or all these other areas where you can majorly find your purpose in life but for a lot of people a good percentage maybe a third or more the job really is fulfilling and is their purpose in life. But it becomes a major stressor as well. Now if it's not your purpose in life. Guess what it can still be your stressor.

So we have to figure out how to get through the day. Enjoy the day and relieve the job stress. I had a great time trading. It was called dealing with difficult people in work and in life. That's a great chapter I think everybody needs. That chapter was one of my most popular chapters. I should do a second one called advanced ways to deal with difficult people in life and in work because the people would grab it up. So I'm going to highly recommend that you figure out how to get rid of the job stress. It may be that you need a different job. It may need an additional chapter. You may need to delegate more. It may mean that you need to take a time management Book. That was another one of my popular Books. So you have to work in the job area and you may need to shift positions.

I remember one time I did a lateral position. I was actually kind of in a downward position but I liked it so much better. My boss was kind enough to let me make the same amount of money even though it was a slightly downward position but I absolutely loved it and it was fantastic. It was good that I went and asked because he would have never given it to me. He would just leave me where I was. He didn't know there was a problem when you're having a problem on your job. You are probably the only person that knows you're having a problem and your job now.

The other great thing that I did in my job is I was constantly trying to figure out ways to make the job more fun. I started having a candy bowl in my office and people are always so happy when I offer him candy. Sometimes if I offered to do something for somebody that made them happy and then I had more buddies at work and it was more fun I would try to come up with a new joke every day. I'd look one up on line and then I would share it with different people at work that made it more fun.

Sometimes I grab some of that candy and if I need a favor from somebody I'd say Hey I couldn't leave you out of this deal I got some candy I want to leave you off a few pieces all by the way if you could expedite this paperwork for me that would be great if they knew I was asking for a favor but I was probably the only person that actually bribed them with candy gave them a little something rather than saying hey I'm gonna give you nothing but could you just expedite this paperwork for me. So it's actually OK to use a shameless bribe like that. At least they got something out of the deal and they're thrilled. I would also give candy to people just to make them happier and that made my job better.

So I tried to figure out as I went through an entire day and I did this for about a week. How could I have more fun at my job? How can I make my job less stressful? I mean it is like a study so I would study it every day. I would take little notes for the day. Put it in a little piece of paper and shove it in my back pocket and then at night I would go through and I would start problem solving and by doing this I was amazed with the creative ideas I came up with in just one week. It felt like I had half the pressure at work the very next week and I had twice as much fun. At least maybe four times as much fun. The very next week. So you actually do have to take the time to write it down on paper. See it in front of you. Problem solve it and then go back and make it happen.

It's just a couple of techniques that you can use to make the job a little bit better. This could be an entire Book right. Just how to make your job more fun, more efficient and more fulfilling. Let's drive on. Let's go to the next one. Now the next major life area is finances. Finances are absolutely huge. Why I once studied it said seventy five percent of marital arguments and we said of the spouse saying happy ain't nobody happy. It was over money. They were money arguments. Can you imagine that? Seventy five percent of everything they ever argued with your wife or your husband was gone.

Why because of the finances. A lot of times it didn't seem like finances. You were arguing about who was going to take the kid to his karate lessons and the real thing wasn't that you had to take him to the karate lessons and interrupt your day and take some of your meat time and go drive home. The thing was Oh now it's gonna cost me even more gas I'm already paying for the karate lessons I got to work extra hours for the karate lessons and now you want me to drive over the karate lessons and if I go with them he's probably going to be testing for a belt he's gonna want 20 bucks from his dad to pay for the belt test and blah blah blah blah blah. Why is this especially visited upon me?

And if he had a million dollars in the bank and you say can you drive the kid to the karate class you don't think about that. You don't worry that you're probably retired because you got a million dollars and you have plenty of free time. He's driving to the class and you're so happy to serve. It's totally different when you have money in the bank. It's kind of an old expression. I'm not sure who said it; it might have been Mae West. It was some kind of famous actress I remember and she said I've been rich and I've been poor in riches. Better money can't buy you happiness isn't exactly true. It can buy a lot of happiness. It can't buy you every kind of happiness but it can buy you an awful lot of happiness. I'll prove it to you.

Notice how much poverty hurts people. You can at least take away that hurt and the opposite of hurt is happiness. OK. When you eliminate the hurt you're free to be happy. Now the other reason to get great finances is so you no longer have to worry about finances. One of the reasons I wanted to have a great career is so I can help a lot of people and B so I can make a bunch of money. Why do I want to make a bunch of money? That's all I could have. Toys and clothes and going on trips and blowing it would be a big shot and all the stuff I could care less about. I want to make enough money that I never have to worry about money again.

The freedom to do what I wanted to do when I wanted to do it and the ability to help others with that extra money in my pocket. A couple of years ago a friend of mine was down on his luck. I was so thrilled he asked me if he could borrow a thousand dollars now a thousand dollars would normally significantly cut into my finances and savings but because I saved up a bunch of money it was really an insignificant amount. I was happy that I had that kind of wealth to be able to help him out. It's actually been two or three years since I even thought to ask him for it. So having those finances is a great way to free up the stress in your life. And I'll tell you when it gets down to the last few dollars man it gets stressful.

So to have good finances you have to learn about finances to study finances. You'd have a financial plan. You have to have a system in place. These are things you have to do. Most people just go out and try to make a bunch of money and hope the finances work out. No it's much more sophisticated that matter of fact retirement even if you put it away like 10 or 20 percent of your income or even 30 or 40 percent of your income maybe half your income you're probably not earning enough that you could actually retire on that amount. You can only retire on that amount if you use the power of compound interest to double it over time. OK.

When it doubles once and then twice and then no time in the near time that's only five or six times and you would have to make what somewhere between you know 30 times as much to three hundred times as much just to come out with the same amount as if you were using the compound interest. This is why it's so important to save early. I think it's about I think there's like a power of 76 you can use as a little formula forget what it is but about say you're making like seven or eight percent about every seven and a half years your money doubles somewhere around that check me on the figures which means if I wait seven years to start putting away money for my retirement I now have to put away twice as much as if I started 7 1/2 years earlier wait 15 years. Now I've got to put away four times as much just to break even with the guy that started 15 years earlier. Now most people don't start saving until their 40s.

It's almost game over which is the probable reason why about 40 percent of the people in the US have to work between now and when they die and a lot of them go bankrupt. But they made more than enough money and people say Oh they blew it on this or that. The other thing maybe they did but they just didn't plan it well and most people just had one too many kids. That's the other financial thing kids are a huge financial burden. They cost about as much as a yacht. They're about a quarter million dollars or more a piece. Now if I said hey I want to go out and I want to have a kid and it'll be fun and we'll make our lives so rich and you know I just always pictured having two or three kids and you just start going out have two or three kids. You say great.

I don't have three kids. If I said OK three kids is the same as I need you to buy three yachts and yachts are three hundred and thirty thousand dollars apiece. So you need to finance a million dollars over the next 30 years. That's a ton of money. That's a ton of money. You don't have that kind of money so high you can do it. It's all going to come out of your retirement. You're going to scrape by going to work tons of extra hours you can have nothing to show for it and then you're going to be 45 to 50 years old and you're gonna have about ten dollars in the bank and you're going to try to retire and you're going to lose and you're going to be one of the great poor. Why? Because you had a medium to small size family.

It's not 1950 anymore and you know just the husband can work and work 40 hours and have you know chicken in every pot and have as many kids as you want. The boss will give you a raise because he knows you have kids and they're going to give you a pension so don't worry about retirement. And at the top of your pension you're going to get Social Security and the wife doesn't have to work. That stuff was true for a very tiny window in American history that lasted about 20-30 years but people still believe it today. And that's why so many Americans crashed. So this whole area of finance you really got to nail down. It's very complicated. Entire nother Book yeah.

Your goals. If you're not moving in the direction of your goals you feel like you're not accomplishing anything. You know why. Because hello. You're not accomplishing anything. I had a dog used to pushing a ball with his nose and he goes zigzagging around the room and I like crazy directions bouncing off the walls. From his perspective he was always pushing the ball forward so he was getting ahead. Now from 10 feet up you could see that he wasn't getting anywhere. He was just zigzagging around. That's what most people are doing like they're like a dog pushing a ball with their nose thinking they're getting the hint.

No you have to have specific plans in place to get a hit on the job. Financially physical goals mental goals spiritual goals any kind of goal you have. The shortest distance between two points is a straight line or resource, a legitimate cheat to get you from here. There you are faster. Your goals have to be written down. You have to have plans. You have to monitor them. You have to adjust them. People need to really set time aside to train on how to achieve goals. This is one of the other things you've been cheated out of. They never taught you this in school.

Even in business school they don't do planning and goal setting and most colleges. I think Harvard and Yale those types of Ivy League schools will actually teach you how to do goal setting and those types of things will teach and do Gantt charts and planning and flow charts and six sigma and all this type of stuff but an average college even the business degree won't teach you how to do these things. It's a shame it's going to determine how you make out in life. So this is just another area that I would go out and I would take some additional chapters. Just a couple hours of a chapter will put you in the top 5 or 10 percent of the country because most people have zero chapters and then they wonder why I failed. How come I didn't get what I wanted. Again you weren't trained now.

Health is a huge area. Remember all the emotions go through the body. This is the only thing carrying you along. You don't want to get to old age and you're old and decrepit yet to your golden years you've worked your entire life. You did save enough money and by the time you are sixty five you're either dead or you're so decrepit you can't really enjoy your life or you're okay when you're 65. But somewhere between 70 to 75 boom now you're sick you're miserable. You have cancer, you've got lung problems, knee problems, back problems, urinary problems, bags hanging off of you urinating in your pants. You know it depends on you. Why do so many people wear alcohol? Alcohol is very rough on your bladder and b poor diet and c lack of exercise so people have leakage because they haven't tightened those muscles.

So it depends on you. It's bad it's the lack of diet and exercise that causes most of the deficiencies. See it's natural to get old and die. It's not natural to get old and sick and die. Matter of fact you should only really be decrepit if a you live to be very old and b just for the last two or three years not from age sixty five to eighty five with twenty years of various illnesses and pains and aches and all these things. Now it should be just as you're getting over the hump right before you're going to die. The last two or three years maybe you have some deficiencies otherwise with a good diet and good exercise. Unless something genetic happens to you or an industrial accident, if you've kept yourself up with a health wise diet and exercise you should do well at old age. It's not a percent guarantee but the best guarantee you can get.

So study nutrition. What do I put in my mouth? I'll give you the mini Book right now. Healthy nature is the least touched by man and the closest to the sun which means fruits first vegetables second than grains then meats. Add in a few seeds and nuts because they're rich sources of life. Boom, you're done. So it doesn't take rocket science a few basic vitamins and minerals. So getting the nutrition part down actually isn't as complicated as people make it. The Health part doesn't have to be as complicated either in terms of exercise. Now here's how you keep yourself up with exercise. It's not that hard. Do a little bit of weight chapter. You need weights to build up the calcium and the structures in your bones. It also keeps the muscles strong. It helps the joints. It helps the ligaments.

The pumping action and lifting action will also work the bile system and clean out toxins and help get blood flow going. Also creating new stem cells in the body keeps you young keeps you youthful, gets your body oxygenated so a little bit of weight resistance chapter then just moving it almost doesn't matter what you do. You can run around. You can go for a jog and go for a walk. You can ride a bike. Just don't be sedentary. Don't be sitting all the time , you don't have to be an Olympic athlete. Just take a walk a couple of times a day. You know, ride a bicycle once in a while. Do a few what I call living room exercises, do a few push ups, do a few sit ups, any muscles that you want to maintain and you want to maintain them all because they all have a function.

So work though so work the abdominals work the legs work the arms work the shoulders. I like yoga because it keeps flexibility. It's the only exercise. At least one of the few exercises that really focuses on flexibility. I also like Taichi because you can do it for the rest of your life. It's a very relaxing, gentle movement you can do between now and when you die. It covers all the major exercise areas. It gives you coordination, it gives you balance. Perfect but just think about some fun things you like to do that are exercise too so playing sports. I like to go for walks. You can do some dancing. You know that's how my wife likes to exercise. She dances in front of the TV or whatever she dances in front of the music box. She just loves to dance. That's how she gets her exercise.

Maybe she overdid it one time at a Zumba class to a dance to do but your boy where she saw the next day. So you have to do it in moderation but have some fun with it. Be active. Move. You know what to do. A lot of times if you have difficulty exercising it's important to take a class because that social aspect I think is great and it motivates you to do it. I don't need other people to motivate me. I need to be easy. So what I did is I took my garage and I made it into a mini gym so I have different pieces of equipment there. I know that I won't pack my stuff up and go all the way to the gym. I know that about myself so I made sure that I just walk down the hall and then I've got a gym there.

Sometimes I'm too lazy to walk down the hall so I've got two pieces of exercise equipment inside my office while I'm reading TV. I've got a couple of free weights and I've got a yoga mat if I want to do some stretching. So even while normally you would be sitting around. I can be stretching and working out a little bit. Moving a little bit on somebody else would just be sitting there for like three or four hours totally stagnant when you're sitting. You have a huge amount of physical atrophy. You've got to be very careful. My job is sanitary.

I sit in front of a microphone and I sit in front of a computer and I talk into the microphone or I tap into the computer. That's not a lot of activity. So all through my day I'm going for walks. I'm hopping on the elliptical machine or my exercise bike. I'm pumping a few weights. I dropped down to do a few pushups. I take the dog for a walk. Maybe I do something in the yard. I might do a few yoga stretches just to loosen up my body during the day. That'll maintain your health. That's it for this chapter. Keep going, you 're doing absolutely fantastic. And I'll see you in the very next chapter.

Assertiveness - Faith - Rules

Hey everybody. here and welcome back. If you were looking for an opportunity to see my smiling face. Here you go. In this chapter we want to talk about how to let go of old pain and how to stop taking in new pain. One of the ways to do that is to be assertive to literally stop taking crap from other people literally handed back to them like I'm doing this picture and say Hey here you go. We need to learn a little bit about assertiveness now. Assertiveness Of course could be an entire Book. I mean do want it in the future but basically assertiveness the definition that I use is acting with skill.

So a lot of people think assertiveness is somewhere between being passive and being aggressive. If you're too passive you get stepped on. If you're too aggressive people get angry at you. But if you're too passive and you're not a serve enough then maybe you need to go up the scale and become more aggressive. That's the way you do it. That can be one strategy. Do it to become a little bit more aggressive but you don't necessarily have to become aggressive to be assertive. So I think of passive and aggressiveness as being on a spectrum like hot and cold assertiveness. I think of it as being related to hot and cold but not the same as temperatures related to hot or cold. But it's nowhere along the spectrum so assertiveness is the same way it's related to being passive and it's related to being aggressive but it's not necessarily on the same spectrum.

So I can be assertive when somebody says something nasty to me. I don't have to be passive or aggressive. I can simply say something like Hey you didn't mean to hurt my feelings when you said that right they'll say Oh no no I didn't mean to do that because these little snipers that tried to snipe at you with these little comments they don't want to be exposed. So that's acting with skill but it's neither passive nor aggressive. But the main takeaway that I want you to get is that you need to learn a little bit about assertiveness if this is a problem area for you.

You can't go through your whole life getting stepped on and the first step just like I'm showing you here in this picture is give it back to him. Here you go. Don't accept it, don't even take it on, think back this way if somebody is being nasty to you and they're being a jerk and people are reading this from the outside they can always spot the jerk. This is why you don't always want to go with the aggressive technique and come back at him. Because if I'm being aggressive towards you and you're being aggressive towards me can you spot the jerk now. No it looks like two jerks going at each other when somebody is being a jerk and you're being good about it then everybody can spot the jerk. They can see that you're just being strong, you're able to take these types of things and the other person is a jerk.

That's a better thing for them to walk away with. But it's even better if you can use a technique like I just share with you to actually use some skill. Now the key core component of this is not to accept the crap that other people are giving you say things like that's your opinion or I don't think that's accurate or I don't accept that or hey you're wrong. I don't ever take crap from anybody. Why? Because I can always be assertive and just hand it back to all, think of it like two people with a tennis ball somebody throws the ball across the net. You can do one of two things.

You can throw the ball back to them which is not taking their crap or you can hold on to the ball and say you didn't mean to hurt my feelings when you said that right. Well now they can't throw the ball back at you because you're holding onto it. S.L. virtually any other way you can win the game so using either technique you'll win the technique you don't want to use is they throw the ball over to you and you start beating yourself upside the head with it which means taking this on. Feeling bad and sitting in it they've only offered you the opportunity to be upset by handing you some crap. You don't have to go to every fight you're invited to. You don't have to own it and you don't have to let it enter you emotionally.

You can simply be assertive and hand it right back to all or use a technique that I gave you and totally take it away from them. Now the next concept I want to teach you is to believe in yourself. Why? Because it's wrong not to, it's absolutely positively insane not to believe in yourself. People have so much self-hate and self-doubt and self regret and self fear you know they're being self-destructive which means you're destroying yourself. That's insane. So I can go out there and I can figure out logically and scientifically and psychologically why somebody else would crap on you because it doesn't hurt them. That actually makes sense.

Sometimes you go out there and you crap on somebody else and you let out your frustration and make you feel better. I can explain why that would be beneficial. Why you crap on yourself. That's insane. That's called self flagellation you're literally beating on yourself thinking that that's somehow going to make you feel better. It's an odd psychological trick that you do when you are a little kid. If you did something wrong or you were bad or you made an error your parents would punish you. So you figured, Well what I'll do psychologically is I'll punish myself ahead of time and then they won't have to do it. That's how screwed up your brain is and don't feel bad.

Almost everybody thinks that way and they don't realize they think that way but that is the only way you can explain why somebody would actually crap on themselves not believe in themselves and make themselves feel bad about themselves. And this is what hurts your self-esteem, not so much what's coming in from the environment and what other people are doing or what's happening out there. It's what's happening inside of you. You simply aren't believing enough in yourself. I want you to take the concept of faith that you should believe in yourself. Why is no one crazy insane? Wrong not to be totally unhelpful. Second reason is you are the only thing you have to work with anyway if you don't believe in yourself. Say well I don't really have tools or skills in this area.

Tools and skills can be learned and you say I did these bad things in the past. Great. Don't do them anymore. Let's judge you on what you do from here forward. I'm telling you if you nail this down if you take some time if you meditate on this. Think about this and reflect on this journal. You can believe in yourself. From here forward start to hear those negative thoughts where you stop believing in yourself. Again examine them you'll see that they're not true. Flush them out and go right back to believing in yourself, shut them down early and often focus on some of the things you have done successfully.

Some of the winds that you've had. Don't focus on the things you've done wrong or the failures that you've had in your life. We've all had those. The whole scientific method is fail fail fail fail fail find the one thing that works and then do that over and over and over again. That's how you become massively successful. Humans do a weird sick thing in their mind where they see fail fail fail fail fail 30 times and only succeed once and they say well I'm only a success one out of three times therefore I'm a massive failure. You do the math completely wrong. The only time that matters is when you succeed. Most of life is trial and error. It's mostly trial and mostly error.

It's only a little bit of success. It takes a lot of tries when you don't know how to do something to be able to do it. I mean that's specifically why I'm doing this Book for you. You don't have to do it through trial and error. You can go right to the answer, you can go right to the tools, the strategies and the technique. Get it right the first time or after just a couple of practices instead of spending months and years and decades trying to figure it out for some people to go from the cradle to the grave from the womb to the tomb and never figure out these things I'm teaching you right here right now. But that does not have to be you. But this piece is so important because if you don't believe in yourself you're not going to work on yourself.

You're not going to value yourself enough to do any of these strategies or any of these techniques. So I want you to believe in yourself the only sane thing to do. Remember the core premise of this chapter was that you were born beautiful, perfect and innocent. It was only covered up. Therefore you can always believe in yourself. You're not bad. You're not wrong, you're not defective, you're perfect. I believe in you. Therefore you should believe in your Here's another great strategy. Don't create rules and pressure. They're only going to end up causing you pain any time you make a rule. You create a boundary, you create something that is going to block you or hurt you. My mom had certain rules about what types of movies she enjoyed.

She likes colleagues because they are funny. She liked documentaries because they were informative and she liked romance and drama because it seemed like it was real life to her and it touched her emotionally. So she liked those movies. Now there were other rules that she had that allowed her to feel bad when there was another type of movie. It blocked her from the enjoyment of the movie because she had a certain rule. She's like well you can't read any violent movies and I mean even violent movies like you know Abbott and Costello or the three stooges where they slap any charge like oh my god that's violence I can't read that. And she would block herself from enjoying it when millions of people had enjoyed it. She wouldn't read science fiction.

Why? Oh my God. That's not real. So therefore you can't enjoy it. She didn't like action movies. Oh it's too much dress, too much tension and guess what there's also violence in it so I'm not going to read that. Well that's like three quarters of all movies now. I didn't have any rules about any of these so I could sit there and read the documentary with her and enjoy it. I go read the chick flicks and enjoy it. I go read the dramas and enjoy it. You know I could read the science fiction ones and the superhero movies and the action adventure movies. I love all the movies. You know I don't limit myself with a rule. I also don't pressure myself anymore about things.

I used to be horrible about being the poster child for just pushing too—hard. It was one of the ways that I motivated myself but I also created a lot of pain for myself. You know I said you're bad and you're not good and you're not this and you're not that I would be so negative to myself if I didn't move in the right direction. I figured that negative motivation would move in that direction. Pretty soon I started associating moving in that direction doing these tasks that would help me accomplish my goal with pain. And guess what. We move away from pain so pretty soon things like going into the gym equal pain. So I moved away from it. I stopped doing things like achieving my life goals going to school start equaling pain going to work start equaling pain you know getting into certain relationships start equaling pain.

Then I started saying no can't you joyously achieve. Can't you feel good you folks and how great you'll feel when you get done with your workout. When you go to the gym can't you just focus on the accomplishments that you're gonna have at work and enjoy each part of the process as you go along. Seeing as one step one micro accomplishment as you go along and enjoy the people around you at work can't you enjoy school. Hey, you're in an air conditioned environment. You're not working out in the hot sun breaking big rocks into little rocks. You're looking at pictures reading the pretty girls go by eating pizzas and haven't followed your friends and you're learning new exciting things. You don't have to pressure yourself to feel good.

Enjoy the knowledge, enjoy the experience, enjoy the air conditioned comfort that you're at. That was different than applying a rule or applying pressure which is only going to cause you pain and remember rules and pressure hurt us and they limit us. People will do rules and relationships. You know you have to respect me. No they don't. You have to respect yourself. But other people don't. Therefore every time somebody disrespects you you're gonna get all upset and you might even cut off that relationship. Hey, maybe they were just having a bad day. Don't set up rules if you don't have to. I used to do this in my dating life with my wife. Thank God she's still my wife because the old rule used to be.

Well you know when you go on a date with a girl you've got to have the flowers and you gotta have the plan and then you gotta have the dinner and then you gotta have the movie and you gotta have all this stuff and everything has to go perfect and has to be just the way I picture it. Otherwise it's a complete failure. Well let me tell you it never comes out exactly the way I pictured hell even when it goes perfect it never comes out exactly the way you pictured. So all these rules were making it painful. So I changed my rule. I said as long as I'm with this girl and as long as I'm with my wife I'm just gonna have a great time. Because we're together and my only rule is I'm I try to make this as much fun as possible for her and I'm going to try to enjoy it as much as I can.

That rule gave me so much more freedom and so much more flexibility. It took 98 percent of the pressure off and the pressure was usually what was causing me to quote unquote failure when a date went bad. I felt so much better. So I want you to think I want you to meditate on where do I create rules and where do I create pressure in my life where I don't need to instead of pressure. How can I create a greater vision? How can I create enjoyment in this process rather than pressure in the rules? How can I loosen the rules or if possible this kind of the platinum standard just get rid of the rules completely. You normally don't need them, you always know the next right thing to do. You don't need a lot of rules in your life.

You know you should work a little harder each day. You know you know you should go on a steady path towards your goals. You know you should always do the next right thing. But we love to put rules in place and allow these rules. What you're going to find is old rubbish, remember the imprint period where you're given all these ideas and those beliefs but they're not really yours. A lot of these old rules allow us old pressures coming from people that aren't you. If something isn't my rule it's something that I'm not pressuring myself about that it shouldn't exist only I should be allowed to myself.

Beginning Coping Skills

OK. Welcome back. Here's another great tool. This will be worth the price of the Book for your right here. It's a way to literally change your self image because a lot of your self image your self esteem is based on the way that you literally describe yourself to yourself so if you say I'm shy. Guess what. You're going to act shy if you say I'm outgoing. Guess what you're going to act out. Now you're saying Hey , I'm a shy guy. I'm a shy gal. I can't just say to myself I'm outgoing and instantly be outgoing. No but you can start to move the needle. You can stop describing yourself as shy and say I'm a little bit introverted OK. I'm a little bit more reflective. That's a better way to describe yourself than shock when the light starts to loosen up a little bit.

You can say instead of being a little bit introverted or reflective I'm a very kind person. I like warm people. I'm warm. I don't jump out there a lot but I'm kind and pleasant. Great. Not much of a leap to go from kind or pleasant to unfriendly. I like people. I like to talk to people. I'd like to make people feel good. Give me an occasional compliment. Just listening to people smile more. That's a gentle leap that you can make, then you could say unkind, unfriendly , friendly means you're a little bit more outgoing, a little bit more active. You can start saying I'm outgoing. I'm not outrageous. I'm not completely and totally energized but I'm an outgoing person. I'm willing to walk up to somebody and say hi and start a conversation.

Do that type of thing you know. And then just keep working your way up the scale. But it's very important that you read how you describe yourself because that's literally going to set your personality in almost like the rules that we talked about the ways you describe yourself like I'm shy as a rule and shy people as a rule have to be what. Very shy. They can be very outgoing. So you're setting up a rule for what you can and can't do by the way you describe yourself. Now you can start to think of yourself as more effective. You can say I don't always get it right. But I always get a result. I learn from everything I do. It's not that I'm a failure. I sometimes have challenges. Sometimes I try things and they don't work but you don't lose until you quit.

So hey I'm not a quitter I'm a fighter. I get out there and I keep doing it until it works. I'm aggressive in that way. These are better ways to describe yourself than seems like I fail an awful lot or I always screw up. Screwing up is how you get to success. It's called a trial. You try something you try. You try to finally hit upon the right solution and then you just repeat that over and over again. That's how all the people that are massively successful do it. It's one of the few ways to learn. There's only two ways to learn. Trial and error. You try to figure it out yourself or what you're doing in this Book called observational learning.

Find somebody who knows what they're doing. Find out how they did it, observe it and then go ahead and try it on your own. Perfect. But this is a great tool. So look at all the different ways you describe yourself because you have a way of describing yourself in virtually every area of your life. You describe yourself in terms of how you feel about yourself. What kind of person you are, what talents you have, what abilities you have, how you judge yourself across a spectrum. Start noticing the words you use to describe yourself and start ticking them up in a positive direction. You will be amazed how transformational this one strategy is. Now I love this technique here. It's a very simple technique to feel better. It's called pet therapy.

There's a strange phenomenon that happens neurologically in your brain when you hang out with your pet, especially dogs they're just kinder, softer they're more interested in you. So this dog you see in the picture here is the absolute perfect dog to use why they're willing to be held. They're soft, they're Fluffy. So you have a chemical known as the love hormone inside your brain called oxytocin. This is the primary one that's released when you hang out with pets. Pets are always kind, always loving, always accepting. So that's a great environment to be in.

But when you stare in their eyes what happens neurologically is you trigger the positive hormones in your system especially that oxytocin and that gets triggered in your system. It also gets triggered in your dog's system. So you start feeling better and they start feeling better. They're looking at you and feeling better. You're looking at them and feeling better and it gets to be this wonderful positive cycle. They found that if you did nothing else in your life but you've got a pet and you had them throughout your lifespan you would add about six to seven years to your life and be healthier along the way. Why? Because pets make you feel fantastic.

Just a quick simple tip: a time you want to feel better simply stare into their eyes. They'll stare into yours. You'll both start feeling better and the dog will actually start liking you better. This is the trick that I did with my dogs. I would do this all the time and my wife's always like how come the dogs like you better than me. Well I know this trick. I look at them more often. They feel love going towards me and seeing my face and feeling love seeing my face and feeling love. They're more attracted to me. So great technique, great tool. Try it out. Helps you instantly feel better now let me ask you a question. Another wonderful picture of me.

I got a little bit of a beard when I worked for myself. So my boss lets me know when is the last time that you actually encouraged yourself. I use the word encourage because the term courage means that you're giving yourself courage when people are discouraging you. The word dis means to remove their removing courage. So you need to encourage yourself, give yourself courage, and feel a little braver about things about asking out the pretty girl or taking a leap or maybe starting your own business or asking for something that you normally wouldn't ask for. Try to encourage yourself to feel good about things. Notice when you discourage yourself and start shutting down those thoughts and then actively try to encourage yourself and start adding in those positive thoughts. It doesn't take a lot to do this technique but it will make you feel wildly different.

It'll boost your confidence significantly. It's so fast, simple and easy to use. Put this on your list of things to do. Now this is an interesting question. I asked this of my therapy clients all the time. I say tell me what's your favorite way to make yourself feel bad. And they go well. When you're feeling bad it's a system you do this then you do this. They do this. They do this and then you feel terrible. So I want you to walk me through your system for feeling bad. So sometimes they're not sure when I say OK. Remember the last time you felt bad. Think about it, get it clear in your mind and then I want you to walk me through the process from start to finish.

What did you do first, second , third and fourth and a lot of times you've gotta walk through how you did it through the different senses so tactically through your body how are you holding your body. How are you breathing? This is all neuro linguistic programming. What was your posture like we were looking up? We breathe in full shadow, shoulders forward, shoulders sunken. What was it? How are you holding your body? How are you moving? We move fast and energized, we are kind of depressed and slow. How are you doing it then? What we are telling ourselves. What types of things are you saying about what you were thinking about what was the inner conversation that was going on. What were the specific things that you told yourself?

Third, what did you picture? What did you imagine? Did you see things going great? Did you see cool and horrible things? How did you do it? How did you get yourself into this specific state? Now this is a great exercise. What do you do with your body? What you do with your words and what do you do with your images, your eyes, so kinesthetic body auditory. Would you say visually they called the Vax system. VK visual way do you imagine this how they do it in neuro linguistic programming. This is what determines your mood. Good, bad or neutral. In this case we're looking for how you do bad. If you do the exact opposite that usually makes you feel fantastic. You can at least stop doing these things and get back in a neutral state which they call serenity.

So realize that when you make yourself feel bad it's not what happens out in the environment it's how you picture it how you handle your body in your words and in your vision that's what makes things so bad. And how you can start to reverse it or at least neutralize it. So realize whenever you're feeling bad this system becomes a good student of your system, interrupts or stops your system and then takes itself in the opposite direction and you'll feel absolutely fantastic. This is a wonderful system. And this one tool alone can literally transform your life. Done correctly. Just take some time. Practice it. Now there's a funny chapter.

You should probably look it up on YouTube. It's by Bob Newhart. It was a little skit. It was called a stop technique and it was done on what they call Mad TV and radio TV was an old TV show I think back from the 90s. And what he would do is he would charge clients five dollars for five minutes and he would do therapy with them and normally didn't go over five minutes and people would tell their problems and he'd say stop it and they'd be what do you mean stop it. He'd say stop it and they go Stop it. Yes. S T O P new word i t. Stop it. It was so funny I showed this in a psychology class and people were roaring but this is a whole theory of psychology.

They don't teach a University called the Stop technique. Once in a while you'll find a self-help book. It's hard to find but the stop technique works great. You start thinking this negative thought oh my mom loved my sister better stop it. OK now I'm going to add in steps to stop it and then destroy it just like we talked about just a moment ago. How do you make yourself feel bad? The stop technique helps you to interrupt it. The second thing is to realize that you have this thought. Figure out all the different ways that this negative thought absolutely positively isn't true. Destroy it. Now if I were to add a third step and I often do. If you want the platinum version to stop, destroy it, replace it. The brain doesn't like a vacuum.

Go ahead and replace it with a thought you want to have the next time this negative thought comes into your head so stop it. That totally interrupts the pattern. Little we say stop it in your head and destroy it. Figure out how it's absolutely wrong. Replace it with a positive replacement for this strategy. If you had no other therapy technique if you want to be a therapist just like Bob Newhart was doing in this little skit and this is all you did you would probably do as well as any therapist out there. Now I'm gonna get letters about this from a therapist they're gonna say no it's not true but given the fact that therapists only have about 20 to 25 percent success rate yes you would have at least a 20 to 25 percent success rate using this one strategy.

Importances" - Forgiveness - Starting Over

Now here's an interesting life strategy for you to reconsider your importance. Now I know importance isn't a real word just considered a -ism but ask yourself Are there certain things in your life that you think are really important that actually aren't. I know a lot of men and a lot of women. They've gotta get their hair and their makeup just right in their outfit just right and they're so worried they think it's so important to just look perfect before they head out the door. But then you spend the whole night worrying about whether or not somebody complimented you or they didn't compliment you.

If you look great. If your hair was just right all night why not just throw on something clean, run a comb through your hair, make sure you shower, make you shave and just head out the door and enjoy yourself. Is it really that important? A lot of times we take small things, we make them huge and they're just not that important. Sometimes an award or a promotion or things like that we get really excited about and they're just not that important in the scheme of things. But we put in so much time and so much energy and here's the kicker. So much of our self-esteem, our self image goes into these things and they're really not that important. Think of it this way: I won two different teaching awards. Now I tell people that because that's a great marketing piece and shows that I'm a good instructor.

But let me ask you a question. Do you think I actually cared about those awards or thought they were important yes and no. I thought it was really nice that my students and the staff thought I was good enough that they gave me that and they wanted to show appreciation. So it's nice to appreciate that part I liked as a Zen philosopher and a Buddhist. I'm looking at this and I'm saying I was teaching at a certain level before they gave me the award and I was teaching at the same level after they gave me the award. It really didn't change therefore the award is meaningless if you're a very vain person. It means a lot if you get it or you don't get it to somebody like me.

I have virtually no ego. It doesn't matter if I get the award or don't get the award I got a second one. It didn't matter if I got it or I didn't get it. You know it just didn't matter because there's no vanity there to be appealed to. It just wasn't important to me, it was more like it was only important as a resume piece. That's about it. So reconsider your importance. Is it really important that you're at 4 percent or 5 percent or 6 percent body fat? Is it really important that you know you go to the gym three times a week or what if you just want once or twice that week you know maybe a double up the next week a lot of people get very intense about falling out of their routines and they get so excited when they feel like they failed because they didn't meet their own standards. Remember these are your standards. You can be off on your standards every once in a while.

There's a lot of people very important to them to have a lot of money so they say well you know I could retire. I got two million dollars but I really want to retire with three million dollars. You say Well that may take another 10 or 20 years of your life. Is it important to retire and have a bunch of money to spend or be able to retire now, spend a little bit less, just a third less but get an extra 10 or 20 years of your life back. For me I'd jump out with two million. You know I'm not sure what the polls are in the audience and what you're thinking but it wouldn't be that important to me to have all the extra toys I'd rather have the extra time with friends and loved ones so always look at and reconsider your importance is especially when they're affecting your self-esteem when they're affecting your moods or they're making you feel bad. Think about it, this one I love.

Forgiveness removes negative thoughts, negative energy removes it from the body, removes it from the mind, removes it from all your muscular tension, and frees up the immune system. Forgiving is not letting the other person off the hook, it's letting you off the hook so that you don't have to live with it so that you don't have this pain in your system. That's why I want people to forgive not because the other person deserves it but you deserve not to have this pain circulating through your system mentally physically , spiritually and emotionally even from an immune system standpoint shortening your life terms of longevity.

So always always forgive and one of the other reasons I want you to forgive others in even life in general for how it may have crapped on you is that if you can forgive others and you can forgive LIFE YOU'LL FORGIVE YOURSELF the mistakes you may remember not forgiving is a philosophy and this philosophy this rule just like judgements if you judge somebody else that will come back and you'll be judging yourself if you don't forgive others then forgiveness is not part of your philosophy. You don't just give it out therefore you won't give it to yourself either. So when you withhold it from others and you withhold that forgiveness from life you're gonna withhold it from yourself. And that alone can destroy your life. Think about what you're forgiving.

It's crap and I say crap. Very specifically because that's literally what it is. It's crap, it's worthless, it has no street value. Your pain has no street value. If I say take a 10 pound bag peg of your pain and go and try and sell it on the street you couldn't even get one dollar for it. That's how worthless your pain is because it's crap. Matter of fact somebody may give you 10 bucks to get the hell away from them. They would want you to walk away with your pain but they will not buy it because it has no value. We do a strange thing psychologically because we quote unquote paid a price for this pain. It costs us something emotionally. We think it has actual value. Your pain has no value. Get rid of it. Say goodbye to bad rubbish, throw it all out.

Say I'm then I'll get rid of all this mental crap. Forgive yourself forgive others forgive. Life. Drive on. Amazingly freeing. You will love it. Now here's what we tell you. Sometimes remember in your conscious mind you can say yes Mr. I'm excited about this. I want to do this. Yes yes yes. Run out there and say I let it all go. I forgave everybody. And you'll feel great but then it'll start to sink back in and you'll start to come back. You know why. Remember your conscious mind can learn things and change its mind very quickly. Your unconscious mind where things reside but they've kind of settled. There's a storehouse of that emotion down there.

It takes a little bit longer. So sometimes you've got to forgive yourself. Others in life. Three times four times 10 times 20 times doesn't matter how many times it takes each time it'll get a little better. Each time a little more will come out of the unconscious and it will truly let it go. So take some time with it. If I do it a few times that's OK it's fine. You do and the technique right. Here's another technique I love. There was an old Bill Cosby skit and he was talking about he remember when you were kids and you went out there and you played stickball and you know maybe you hit a ball right down the line and kids were arguing you know it wasn't on this side the line wasn't on that side of lie and what you would finally do is you would say to hell with it and say do over and all kids agree on that.

They say do over. OK you know throw the ball to again see what happens this time maybe hits it maybe goes in maybe goes out but at least we'll know one way or the other do over. A lot of us in life could use a do over. Here's the interesting thing. You can actually as a philosophy and in reality start your life over again any day any moment that you decide and say OK. There's a dividing line in my life from here forward I'm going to move forward. I've done this several times in my life. I even started keeping a journal at one point when I was around 25 to 30. Somewhere there I started keeping a journal.

And if I decided I was going to start a new dividing line in my life I would post that in my journal or I would start a new journal. It was like literally a new chapter was a fresh Word document that I would use and I would start a new chapter and I would say today is the first day the rest of my life read a little corny but you know you put something like that or today my life begins anew. This is the dividing line. So it was very clear black and white in print in her eyes. I looked back through my journals and I could see the progress so I know that no matter how bad your life was or if you just want to go on to the next great adventure and start doing things differently you can say today is the dividing line in my life.

And jump in. I'll tell you a little story. There was a lady in my master's class. We were having what they call a culminating experience. We were kind of having our last day of classroom time in one of the classes that we did was just a round robin. We were literally talking about what we wanted to do with the next five years of our life. Why we got into the program, what we thought we had accomplished and what we want to do next. Well it came to this lady and I'm thinking that she's kind of a little old to be in the master's program because she must have been like sixty five. She might be a little older than that but let's say sixty five.

She said Well you know what. I had a horrible childhood and I was abused and there was this going on and that was that going on in my life was just horrible. And I never got over it. So these are things that happened between the time she was like you know a newborn until she was maybe like 12 years old. She stayed in that pain for the rest of her life. And then she said Well I went I got a bachelors and I said well if I get a bachelor's degree in psychology then I'll be able to figure out how to fix my life. And then I can let go of this pain and then I can move forward with my life. This will be great. She got the bachelors and it helped a little bit but barely took the edge off of it.

She still had all this horrible pain she was still very much fixated on her past in literally wrapping herself in rolling over and over again in this pain rehearsing it in her head totally immersed in her past. Then she said well I'll go and I'll get the masters. The Masters surely will have the skills that I need. And she said I'm kind of disappointed. I don't want to say anything bad about the university but I did everything I could. I read books on the side. You know I tried to figure it out and I still haven't figured out how to get rid of this old pain. All the pain is just following me. It's haunting me. It colors everything I do in my life. I still feel absolutely terrible and I said to her Here's a great technique for you to do over. Just start your life again and go from here forward and leave everything in the past behind.

Just start again. And she's like she was deeply offended. She's like so indignant Oh my God you can't just do that. I'm like No no no you don't understand. I'm not asking you if you can do it or you can't do it. I'm asking you if you will do it or you won't do it. You know why. Because I've already done it. I've read that hundreds of people start their life over again. I'm not asking if it can be done. I'm asking you if you're going to do it. Well she just maintained her defensiveness and she was upset about this and this was just the stupidest thing you ever heard. So guess what. She's probably still living with her pain. She's one of those people that had a lot of faith in their problem and no faith in themselves.

They defended themselves from every solution which was the probable reason that they maintained and still have the problem today because they wouldn't get this one concept that you can start your life over any day you want from a Zen perspective. They don't care what you think. Each day is a fresh new day. You can never relive even one second of the past. From a Zen philosophy you are forced to restart your life over again every single day. And that's not a bad thing. That's a beautiful thing. Today is a fresh new day totally untouched totally Virgin totally pure wonderful day to have the experience of life. That's the Zen philosophy. So I leave you with this philosophy. You can make the dividing line your life start over any time you want.

The past isn't getting any better. You don't want to do a lot. I know a lot of therapists love this. They'd love to have you go in the past and they'd love to have your role in it and go back and forth and do all this and make all your amends and clean everything up. Sometimes it's better just to cut bait and go forward. Yes, maybe you should go back and do some amends. I like that little piece. But you don't have to try to make yesterday better. They call the past the perfect preservative if it was great. It's over. If it was horrible it's over. Remember there's a quote in the book that said this power is denied even to God the ability to change the past.

So no matter how much you talk about it, do therapy on it whatever you did in the past and get any better. So the people that did the best in therapy with me are the people that were willing to start over and say you know we're going to take all this debt this psychic debt away and you're just going to start at zero and go forward with better instructions with better tools with a better attitude and things are better now and they're just gonna keep getting better. Let's do that. And those people in therapy did absolutely fantastic. So that's my wish for you to make it happen. Jump in. Fantastic technique. This is worth the price of the Book alone. Use it.

Growth - Self Evaluation - Letting Go

Here's another great self-help technique for you. Do one thing each day to make your life just a little bit better. The accumulation of these efforts is going to make a huge difference over time. It's like compound interest upon compound interest. They say small steps repeated can accomplish any undertaking. So one small thing each day isn't so small in a few weeks, a few months or a few years. I used to tell my therapy clients here's kind of where you are in life. If you could survive things getting worse and worse you could survive things getting better and better. And now that you've had this chapter that's where you are in your life. Things are gonna get better and better and better all depending upon how much you use these strategies and techniques and what level you're willing to take it.

But the least you can do is do one thing each day just to make your life a little bit better. Literally like you see the plants here. Plant the seeds to let that slow accumulation happen. If you accomplish one thing each day even if you have a loss you say well I had a loss over here but I also had a gain over here and this thing is going to grow over time. The loss is just finished. Whatever it was , it's not going to get any bigger. It's done. But this small gain can grow. And today wasn't a complete loss because I gained one thing. I used to say no day is a loss. If I learned one thing so every day I made a goal to read at least one page or at least I got to a spot where I took a note.

There was something that I learned there that I thought enough to circle it or highlight or start or put a little note next to it, something that I could do to make my life a little bit better. If you buy decent books you probably don't get more than a page into it before you find at least one thing like that. So do one thing each day to make your life better and you'll start to feel fantastic and not just feel fantastic. Your life is going to start to go fantastic. I love this technique because it brings back an old great memory that I have when I was bowling with my dad. I felt like I was a big shot because he was going to let me keep score that day so I felt like I was a big dog.

So we're bowling along and we're having a great time and I'm keeping the score and you know I couldn't believe it when I looked at the scoreboard and I said Oh my God I'm actually beating my dad I'm doing fantastic. And he looked it over and he said Oh you made a little air here and you made a little air here. He said Good news bad news. The bad news is you're not that great a bowler but the great news is you keep score fantastic. You heard of an awesome scorekeeper. So this is kind of where I learned the analogy that sometimes we're winning in life but we're just keeping score lousy. We're doing the opposite of what I was doing. We're actually winning but the way we're keeping score actually makes it look like we're losing.

You're better off using the system I use rather than a little kid. I was kind of losing but I felt fantastic because it looked like I was winning based on the way that I kept score. So you need to re-evaluate yourself to give yourself a higher score. How did you do? And a lot of times were not even it's not even giving yourself a higher score giving yourself more credit for the good things that you do. Sometimes we're not evaluating properly. Sometimes you go out on a date with a girl and you say oh you know or a guy and you say oh I did terrible on that day but maybe the date went lousy but it wasn't you. Maybe it was actually. Then I can date a girl one time and I say oh it didn't go that good because I didn't feel like we really connected.

And she wasn't really into me and I didn't feel really good about the date. I didn't feel like I performed well. And you know I don't know if I want to go out with her again or if she doesn't. She may not feel like she wants to go out with me again. It just went horrible. Well that's one way to look at it the other way to look at it is to go through and analyze the date and say what went right and what went wrong. And I started from my end and I said well I picked her up so I was willing to travel to her. She didn't travel to me, I traveled to her so I can score myself high. They're certainly way higher than her. She did nothing. So far I've done everything. Then I opened the door for her and I was very kind to her and complimented her and I brought her some flowers. Win win win.

I'm doing fine. There's nothing that I'm doing wrong yet. I took her out for a meal. I paid for everything. You know, we even went out for coffee afterwards. I paid for the fact that she didn't offer to pay for anything and that's OK. So I'm doing great. I tried to encourage her about things and talk about positive things and do a lot of good listening and those types of things. And I was very kind to her. I didn't pressure her for a kiss at the end of the night I just kind of gave her a hug and off she went on our way. So I did very well and I said to God, "Why was the date such a disaster?" And I went through what she did and I scored her and I said Yeah I had to drive to her because she never on any of these dates ever drives to me.

I always pay for everything she won't even once in a while pick up a cup of coffee. Most girls do that; they'll spend five bucks if you spend fifty for a meal or something. They'll do that just as a kindness or buy an ice cream or something once in a while. She never does that. Isn't that strange. I was very complimentary of her but she criticized several things about me. That was kind of odd. And then I gave her a hug. She didn't come and hug me. She wasn't being very kind or loving. She wasn't showing any affection. I would reach over and maybe hold her hands and make her feel good and look in her eyes and do these types of things.

She wasn't doing that back to me. So the reason I didn't feel connected is she was doing a lousy job of connecting. She was doing a lousy job of reciprocating. She didn't really bring any value. Actually as I look back over it and I looked over two or three dates that I had with this girl I said wow we've had one two three three dates and she didn't add any value to any of those dates. He really didn't do one positive thing but I was so worried I was so controlling, feeling like I can control everything from my side. I can make this disco great and therefore if I'm controlling it the date doesn't go great. Then I failed. Now I can actually fail from the other side.

And quite often does. So I was keeping score on these dates lousy and thinking Man I must just be so uninteresting so boring so not this so not that you know all these things and really in the day I said wow it's really her. I'm not kidding myself about this. I also looked at how it could not be her, how it could be me and I couldn't come up with anything. No it was pretty much her that was an accurate fair assessment but I totally thought it was me until I did a better more accurate more detached analysis so a lot of times in life we're not evaluating ourselves fairly or high enough. It's one of the weird things that you do psychologically: you try to score yourself lower and be very conservative. That way you're not overestimating your abilities and that can be a protective factor in life. You know you think you'll do OK but you end up doing great.

And even if you don't do great you end up doing OK is a good thing I didn't overestimate myself. That's a protective factor but boy is that lousy for your self esteem. So that's the reason why your brain does that. But it's one of the things that hurts your self-esteem. The mis evaluation is the other thing that hurts it. You weren't looking at who was doing what. And giving proper credit where credit was due. Or maybe you were looking at it wrong. I was always looking at it from my perspective. What did I do right or wrong? I should have looked at it from the other side and said Well every relationship no matter how thin you slice it there's always two sides. How would you score her if you gave her the same criteria?

So even getting the philosophy of how I score myself right can sometimes be difficult. This is a very important area. Virtually everybody has low self-esteem. We'll have an issue in this area in virtually every human being where they have probably self esteem or not. Does this in some way shape or form if you have fantastic self-esteem? It could have been super duper fantastic if you didn't do this. It always knocks you down. So that's that technique. Use it, evaluate it, play with it to do fantastic things and make you feel so much better and let me ask you a question. What pain are you holding onto a lot of times? The problem is that we've had pain in our lives. The problem is that we're holding onto it and we loop it in our mind.

Think of it this way somebody walks up to me and they call me a jerk. Hey you're a jerk. One two maybe three seconds tops so I can blame them for those three seconds and it's absolutely positively their fault. I can line up people that saw that event and say whose fault do you think that was. Was this guy mean to and they'll say absolutely that was his fault it wasn't yours he was me great I blame for those 3 seconds. Now I think about this thing a thousand times in the next week. Three thousand seconds are my fault. Three seconds is he who is really doing you know ninety nine point ninety nine that I got three decimal points nine nine nine percent of the damage point 0 0 1 percent the jerk ninety nine point nine nine nine percent me and let me ask you another question.

Not only what pain are you holding onto. That's really what's hurting you. Think of it like somebody handed you a hot rock that would do limited damage if they put it in your hand you immediately dropped it. You have a little burn or a little rash or something but it wouldn't be that bad. Now if you keep holding on to it eventually you can lose the whole hand. Right. It'll keep burning and burning and burning. The fact that they put it in your hand is their fault. The fact that you held on to it is yours. The thing that's doing ninety nine point nine nine nine percent of damage is you holding onto it. Let it go. So that's my second question. You must have some kind of timer if you're holding onto it. Some people hold onto things for a few minutes, a few hours, a few days, a few weeks, a few years.

Some people hold on to it for decades and some people say if you offended me I hold onto that forever between now and when either you or I die. Sometimes even they can die and they still hold on to it. It's until I die. That's not a good timer especially because we're making up basically rules. When is it okay to let this go? I'm going to tell you it's okay to let it go immediately. It's OK. Not even to let these painful things in. Somebody calls you a jerk and you go oh how sad they're having such a bad day that they have so much pain in their life they have to spray it on others. I don't even let it get inside of me.

At least half the time when it does get inside of me I say when would be a good time to let it go and I let it go pretty quickly. I kind of feel that having the experience of flushing it out of my system has no value to me so I don't hold on to it. I let it go and off it goes into the universe never to burn me again. Why do I do that? Because I've used the system that you're probably still using which is to turn it over and over and over and over and you had hope and yesterday changes or it gets better or you just burn it out. You hope that goes away. They say time heals all wounds.

Now it just continues to wound you over and over and over again. Let it go. Decide for a very short period of time. That would be a good time frame to feel it and let it go. Maybe a couple of minutes, maybe a couple hours, maybe a couple of days. Don't go into weeks and years and just let it go. You will feel so much better looking back through your own pain, taking something small and working your way up and saying. I'm still holding on to this. Yes. Will we'll be a good time to let it go. Now in practice letting it go. And remember sometimes you gotta let it go a few times because you're unconscious a little slow but let it go let it go let it go so letting it go is an art form in one you need to really learn, study and then practice there's a lot of different ways to let it go. Bruce Lee you used to take his resentments. He'd write them down on a piece of paper. He crumpled them up and then he'd burn them and imagine that they were gone. And if you believe that's true it will become true for you.

My kung fu instructor said that negativity in the martial arts is considered an energy for somebody who's transferred some negative energy. You accepted it. Therefore it got inside of you. You picture it like a negative energy maybe in your center maybe new Che maybe in your heart you picture that ball of energy you put it out into your hands you collect the ball in front of you and then you picture the ball drifting away now from a mysticism point that works perfect psychologically because it's scientifically because you're imagining it you're giving yourself a visual rechapter you're imagining it going away just like it worked for Bruce Lee it will work for you so it's almost an infinite number of ways to let things go. The key is just to find a system that works for you and then use it over and over and over again and you will do absolutely fantastic.

Beating Stress - Guilt & Worry - "Explanatory Style"

OK here's a great new technique for you. This one I call the genius of Alcoholics Anonymous. I was told that the genius of the Big Book of Alcoholics Anonymous was that it had two kinds of stories in it. Here's the stories about people that failed. If you'd do what they do you'll very likely fail. There was another set of stories. If you do it this person does that successfully and you duplicate it. You'll very likely succeed. So I think this is what we need to do in our life. We're looking at our anxiety or depression or bad relationships, our low self-esteem and all these different issues. We need to notice what makes us feel good, what makes us feel bad, and what makes us feel good. Less of what makes us feel bad.

We also need to notice what's working in a relationship. Is this actually moving in the direction I want to go? Or is it taking me further away. Notice what works. Do less of that or eliminate completely and do more of what does work. That's what they call a genius. The Big Book by simply doing those two things even if on a scientific level on a complicated level and a sophisticated level as any kind of level you can think about. You don't know why this works. It'll still tend to work. About 98 percent of the time. Why? Because when you duplicate a system whether it's success or failure and you duplicated well it tends to come out the same.

So we need to be good students of our lives, figure out what's working and maybe even some ways that we can work it a little bit better and do that and eliminate everything that doesn't work now in the same vein. I want you to notice what stresses you. And then learn how to beat it. So make this like your To Do list. If you say Boy I've had anger management problems and my kids are driving me nuts and I have problems coping with different things. Great. Get a Book on anger management parenting and coping skills. Perfect. When we say everything is first to study and then practice well before it's a study you have to do an assessment. Figure out what areas I really need to be working on.

So take the Books, do the self-help books but notice what's stressing you and do the same thing that I just mentioned. When you have a challenge in one of these areas, notice what works. Notice what doesn't work. Eliminate the things that don't work and spend more time with the things that do you'll do fantastic now going to teach you a great therapy technique. It's called sentence stem completion and all you do is put in your version your ending of a sentence so I say one thing I could do to be less stressed would be dot dot dot. You fill in the blank and you go down with a piece of paper and you write one thing I could do to reduce my stress and then finish it again and again and again.

Now the further down you get I think in some ways the more brilliant the answers become because you're not putting down your standard answers your standard answers are probably the first three to five things that you put down the things that are unique that maybe you haven't really focused on haven't really tried before will be numbers six seven eight nine ten might be all the way down to number 20 but at least you will have a good list of things that you can do to help you with your stress your anxiety your phobias your low self esteem whatever it is this is coming from you not from me from you in some ways I think your unconscious mind will help you with this and all of a sudden you'll come up.

with new ideas I highly recommend that you say this sentence stem completions because once you fill them out if you leave them alone for a little while you say boy I can't think of one more thing but then you look at the next day and the next day and the next day on one of those days a piece of genius is going to hit you again this is probably your unconscious bubbling up and you're going to think of one more answer or another answer or you'll be reading something or reading something or bring something to mind say oh I could use that to help me with this sentence then completion this challenge in my life that may be a new solution that I never thought of.

So this is not only going to give you a list of different ways you can help yourself but it's going to activate your particular activator that scans the environment because you focused on something to find more solutions. I've seen people do great therapy using nothing but sentence stem completion. Why? Because you can use it in virtually any area of your life. Think of all the different areas one way I could be a better parent is to one way I could connect with my child more is to one way I can lose weight is one way I could boost my finance is if I were being completely honest with myself I would begin to realize see that was not a solution one it's an insight one one thing I'm trying to push out of my mind is that's an insight one so there's insight ones and there's solution ones.

So ask yourself different styles of questions you know and go ahead and finish out those sentences. I used to use this with clients who said oh I don't know how to solve my problems. I can't think of one thing that I could do to make this any better. And then I'd kind of look at them a little funny and I'd say hey let's try something Let's try a sentence stem completion exercise. And I was always impressed with the brilliant ideas that they would come up with. And I'll tell you a little trick in therapy if you come up with a solution instead of me you're much more likely to follow through. And it makes you feel a lot smarter. So usually if I pushed people to go at least 10 down and their sentence stem completion they would come up with a technique or something close to it that I was going to give them anyways. And I'd say Hey I really like number seven. I would tweak it a little bit like this but I think it's brilliant that you came up with that.

And then I would give him some advice about how to move forward and how to do it. Why? Because that's what I was going to come up with anyways so sentence completion is a great tool. Use it. Try it, see what you come up with. I think you'll be very impressed with what you come up with. Now exercise we've talked a little bit about this before but it's a very powerful mood boost. Remember he said it had about a 25 percent success rate. It worked about as good as the psychotropic meds and worked great with the psychotropic meds but it also does some other things. It relaxes the muscles it pushes out while it gets you focused. That's why it's such a great stress reliever. So there's muscular relaxation, there's endorphins going on but above and beyond all that.

Most people don't think of this. Most of your bad mood negative self-esteem anxiety depression all these types of things that are bothering you is because you're thinking too much you're focusing on your problems when you are exercising you're focusing on what exercising especially if you're chapter really hard or have to practice balance or timing or flexibility or you're lifting a really heavy weight or really pushing yourself. You have to focus on this one thing especially if you're in an exercise class and you have to follow the instructor you're only going to be thinking about exactly what you're doing. That kind of getting out of your head is absolutely fantastic for your mental health and can help you in a ton of different areas. And your brain is always saying "Why am I doing this?"

Well if you're exercising you're trying to make yourself feel better, look better and be healthier. It must mean you really like yourself. I'm going to tell you that it's great for your self-esteem and it's great for your overall mental health. And just having a routine like exercising if you do it on a regular basis can also be very firm and steadying. It gives people a foundation of guilt and worry. I call these useless emotions. What happens is there's functional guilt and functional worry then there's dysfunctional guilt and dysfunctional worry guilt and worry are supposed to be signals when you feel guilty or a little worried about something. It's supposed to trigger you if you're feeling guilty that you should look at what you did examine it.

Think about how you would do it differently if you could do it again and how are you going to correct it. Apologize makeup. Commit an act whatever you need to do. So you feel guilty. You recognize the problem. You come up with a solution and you take action. That's functional guilt. Why? Because it solves a problem. Dysfunctional guilt is almost the same when you notice something that you feel guilty about. You come up with a solution. You take action but then you keep feeling guilty at that point. Dysfunctional. You're supposed to have let it go. Here's another former dysfunctional guilt you feel guilty you feel so guilty you never take an action and then you feel guilty for the rest of your life.

Also dysfunctional Gail uses guilt and worries the way they're supposed to be used. Warrior works the same way it's supposed to draw your attention to an area that needs attention. It's supposed to create an action that is supposed to motivate you to take an action not you worry so much you hide from the thing that's dysfunctional worry but functional worry where you worry about it you analyze it you come up with a plan. You take care of it and then you let the worry go. Why? Because you've done everything that you can't so those are the useful ways of using guilt and worry. And you can also see the dysfunctional ways to use it the right way. Don't use it the wrong way and guilt and worry will almost evaporate as an issue for you see them as signals now. I want you to change what's called your explanatory style.

Let me show you what that is. Because this is absolutely huge in changing the way you feel everybody has what we call an explanatory style. You can see it right in the word. It comes from the root word explain. It's literally our way of explaining things that are going on around us or things that we're doing or how we feel about things. So our ways of explaining things are going to determine what we will do, what we won't do and how we'll feel. We seem to be very cautious. Say I ask a pretty girl out and she says no I don't think so if I explain that as I'm ugly I'm a loser I'm not good enough girls don't like me I screw this up I should have done something different you know all these different things and they're not true that explanatory style is going to make me feel terrible and it could be entirely the wrong explanation. She might be gay. I don't know.

You could be right. She could be dating somebody else and she should say no I just didn't know she was dating somebody else she could be married. OK she could be on a spiritual retreat she could be celibate. I don't know. Maybe I'm just not her type. Doesn't mean I'm not somebody else's type. I'm just not her type. There's no judging for that. There's nothing wrong with me. So a lot of times what we do is we immediately go for the negative when we're explaining things our brain thinks that's protective but really all it is is negativity. So look at the way that you explain things to yourself. We talked about this earlier in another example. Did you have a failure? Or did you get a result?

Maybe this quote unquote failure shows you one more way not to do something. So you try something different, you try something different, you're going through a process of elimination, find the one way that works and then use it over and over and over again. Beautiful that's how all massive success happens but if you just explain it to yourself Oh I lost once I lost twice I lost three times I should just quit. That probably does make you into a loser you know don't go that route. Be careful how you explain things to yourself. When I look at how depressed people explain things to themselves, guess what. They do it in depressing ways things are never gonna get any better. This always happens to me. I'm such a loser.

Blah blah blah blah blah. They've always got a negative way to describe the situation themselves in the future. The Optimist does the exact same thing but they have a different explanatory style. I failed once but I'm not done yet. Oh good. I'm getting a little closer to the correct answer. Great. I know if I try this X number of times but eventually I'll hit it. I know today was bad but hey now I've hit bottom. So tomorrow will definitely be better. The optimist has a much better way of describing things I can remember when I used to be the pretty girl out. She would say no. I would always figure there was something wrong with me. My buddy Nick would always say hey best she never had and drive on. Realizing she must have had poor taste or you go back to my original analogy. Probably just wasn't a match.

He was playing a numbers game. He didn't even care. He would line up three or four different women; his average was 50-50. So he figured if he lined up for he's going to get somewhere between 1 and 4 dates. Very rarely would he strike out four times and if he did because he lined up so many he was still OK. I had a worse system. I'd look at a girl and get all excited about a girl. I get nervous about a girl and then I'd wait and I'd wait and wait. Then I'd finally ask her out and if I ever got stung because she said no man I'd be another six months for another look at another girl again. At least in terms of asking her out. Nick sat me down and said no no it's a numbers game and said all the right people will say yes and all the right people will say no you know.

Very rarely is somebody confused. So it's just a numbers game. So how we describe things to ourselves and how we explain things to ourselves is absolutely huge. If you did nothing but this changed the way you describe things to yourself I can almost guarantee you that about seventy five to eighty five percent of your anxiety, your low self esteem, your depression and virtually almost any disorder that you have any kind of mental pain or challenge you have will get significantly better. This is at the heart and the core of why you feel so bad and why you have old pain. Sometimes your explanatory style is even partially a belief system once something happens. I explain my self explanatory style. This lasts forever.

The classic thing is like sin in the church. OK. If you do a sin well God may forgive you. But when you go to see St. Peter's at the gate he keeps score. He's got a little pad Oh took the Lord's name in vain X number of times you didn't love your neighbor blah blah blah blah blah. Forgot to feed the dog.

All the negative list that he goes through is the positive list but nothing ever goes away. That's one way of explaining things in life but it's not probably the most positive way to do it. So how you explain things is huge. Listening to yourself talk the way you talk to yourself in your head, the things that you say to yourself in the ways that you describe now , explanatory style also has a lot to do with the words you use. OK.

Do you say I lost that time or I'm a loser. Lost in loser sounds about the same but in terms of intensity they're wildly different. I was upset versus I was enraged. This is horrible versus this is bad. Just changing that language a little bit. We do this a lot. Neuro Linguistic Programming. Check out that Book of my neuro linguistic programming and LP. The language that you choose is part of your explanatory style and they have different emotional content so look at how you explain it and then the word choice and you will have this nailed.

Life Is Hard" - Responsibility -
"Dirty Secret Of Psychology"

Now, this concept relates to Buddha's first noble truth that life is suffering. Life is hard. So in this coping skill, what you're doing is once you realize life is hard. Once you get rid of the illusion that it shouldn't be hard, you don't worry about it anymore. If you don't expect to go out and shovel manure every day, then shoveling manure is hard. If your boss says, Hey, I want you to get out of your air conditioned office, pull your chair out, get up from your desk, walk outside, go in the hot sun and shovel manure. You will think life is exceptionally hard and you should never be put through that. And if you've got to do that day in and day out, you're probably going to go back out and shoot yourself.

Now, if you grew up on a farm, you would go out and you would shovel manure every day and say, Of course I shovel manure. This manure won't shovel itself. Why would I ever get upset about shoveling manure? Maybe not my favorite task of all the tasks on the farm, but I really don't care that much. It just needs to be done. So I do it. What's your question? So accepting those things which are hard in our life makes them far less difficult. It's a great philosophy. Now, the second reason we think life is hard is we think these things shouldn't happen to us. They call that and repeat. They call that shooting on yourself. I heard of one comedian. He said, It's rough out there. You better wear a cup. Why? Well, I'll tell you what a business author I read said.

He said life is going to come by when you're in business and it's going to kick you right between the legs at least once a day, sometimes two or three times a day. It's an amazing day when it doesn't happen at least once, but once or twice, maybe three times. That's about the average. You're going to have problems in the business and these things are going to come by and kick you right between the legs. Don't feel bad about it. Don't think this is especially visited upon you. This just tells you one simple thing. Hello. You're still in business. This is supposed to happen. The people that whine and—and complain say, Oh, these horrible things shouldn't happen.

And you know what? Philosophically, maybe you're right. Maybe I was a good person. You walk a little old lady across the street, Maybe these things shouldn't happen to you. But guess what? They're going to that problem will only go away when you go bankrupt and your business goes away. Or hopefully it won't be. Then it'll be when you retire. But between now and then, it's going to happen. Just plan on it. Now what doesn't have to happen is you feeling bad about it for long periods of time. So like I've shared in previous chapters, if you're a fan of , I think I'm up to about 20 chapters now and growing. I've told you before that you have a problem, you feel bad about it, and then you solve the problem.

It's a three step process. But one of those steps isn't necessary. Let's go through it again. You have a problem. You feel bad about a problem, you solve a problem. Can you spot the unnecessary step? Yeah. It's the one right in the middle.

Feeling bad about the problem. And if you do feel a little bad about it, how long should you feel bad about it? 5 minutes, Five days, five weeks, five years? Forever. Which one is it for? You? Keep it short or just eliminate it entirely. In the big book, they say, When I stop focusing on the problem and I start focusing on the solution, the problem disappears. One of the ways to get past these challenges is to immediately go from problem focused. Oh my God, this is horrible.

This is happening to me and get right into the solution. One that'll take it off your plate quicker so it's not sitting in your hand like a hot coal. And two, it completely shifts the focus and you'll feel better knowing that you're getting rid of it versus kind of saturating it, soaking in it, marinating it, just sitting there staring at the problem. Get rid of it fast. You'll feel so much better. Great technique. Now the word responsibility is an interesting word. I kind of split it into response ability, your ability to respond as you gain more. These tools that I'm sharing with you, you have a higher level of response ability. You're able to respond in more ways and in better ways, and sometimes maybe putting a couple of techniques together in more synergistic ways and your ability to respond is vastly improved.

That's why your life improves, because the quality of your response to life is changing, improving. You're learning new tools, new strategies, new techniques, new philosophies, new ways of looking at things, new ways of being in the world. This is awesome. Now, when it comes to straight up responsibility, the classic use of the word. If you take too much responsibility, you're going to hurt yourself. Y you're being literally overly responsible. So the old Zen philosophy is too much of something not good, too little of something not good right down the middle. Perfect. So when you take on too much responsibility, you're taking on too much pain, too much guilt, too much, maybe even authority. You're taking on too much. Too much. Back it off a little bit.

You can still get it done without marinating in it, feeling bad about it, and feeling overly responsible. Take the right amount of responsibility and just solve it. So again, you've got a problem and you solve the problem. Now you don't want to take too little responsibility and say, Oh, that's not my fault. That's not my thing. If you take too much responsibility, you feel bad, you feel guilty, it drains your energy. If you take too little, then you don't take enough action. You don't own up to things and people see you as small or as somebody that whines,—and complains. That's irresponsible. That's not a great word. Right.

And doesn't take action, doesn't actually solve things. And that will make your life go to hell pretty quick. So taking on too little responsibility is probably worse than taking on too much, but you want to do just the right amount. I love this one. Life is too serious to take too seriously. Me and my buddy Nick, we used to have an expression. You can laugh about it or cry about it. Certain things. We started to think that when things went to hell in our lives, the worse it was, the funnier it was. Because at some point these problems just got ridiculous, you know? And we decided you could laugh about it or cry about it. So we thought it was funny that the other person was having this problem. We thought it was funny that it was the other person's turn.

When we tell each other our problems, we try to figure out what was funny about this situation. And because we took it lighter, it freed up our mind. Remove the tension. Tension and pain cause mental blocks. When you laugh about something, you can get past it. It frees up your mind, and then you start coming up with great solutions. Any have more energy as you go out there to actually deal with it. Some people just get so uptight, so focused on things. They tighten up, they tighten up their mental resources, which means cut them off, that they can't solve the problems or become so much harder to solve the problems. It just gets ridiculous.

Don't take things too seriously. It's almost like the deathbed scenario. Are you going to care about these things on your deathbed? Me and Nick used to always say, You know, 100 years from now, who's going to give a—? Nobody. So it puts things in the right perspective. So not taking life too seriously means putting things in their proper perspective whenever possible. Have a good laugh about it, but don't sit there and cry about it. Or if you're going to cry about it, you know, have your angst, get through it, get over it, and then get on with it. Remember life is too serious to take too seriously. I try to have fun with everything, even my problems. Me and Nicky used to look at it in terms of buying time. Somebody else is finished complaining about this. We'll have it solved.

That was one of our literal philosophies. They will freeze like deer in the headlights when they see the problems. They're going to want to sit around and—about it. They're going to whine about it, they're going to complain about it. And maybe if it becomes painful enough later, if they think it's their responsibility or they can get brownie points for it, maybe, maybe, maybe they'll take action. That's a horrible way to do it. Me and Nick would be like, I'll bet you between the two of us and Nick, we can kick this out in like an hour. And you go, Yeah, And we jump in and we would kick it out. Now, if I came back a week later, most of those people would probably still be complaining about it.

We like to see ourselves not as whiners,—and complainers, but people that kick butt and take names. So we loved it when a good problem came up because we thought it would be impressive that we solved something that was this high, a level of problem, and that we did it with grace, which means not whining, not—, not complaining, good positive mental attitude and just kick it out. Not Pollyanna, not pie in the sky, just refusing to hurt ourselves about something that was already hurting us and taking joy in making that problem go away for ourselves and for others. Great philosophy. Now I'm going to teach you one of the dirty secrets of psychology. I want you to know that you're not alone. Everybody is horribly flawed.

What do I mean by that? Your brain is damaged. Everybody has brain damage. There are built in defects in the human brain. Uh, you're studying this Book. I can tell you almost exactly how much of this Book you're going to remember.

And that's assuming you're paying relatively good attention. About 4%. It's one of the defects built into the human brain. The human retention rate is right around 4%. You read 100 words. You remember about four of them. That is really, really low. That's why people have to repeat things over and over and over again. Now, you may say, Oh, I don't believe that, Mr. .

I remember so much more. Well, there's fluctuation, but on average, a human being, it is going to come in at 4%. Here's how you can test it if you don't think it's 4%. Take 200 words and try to memorize them line by line and see how many times you have to go over it to remember more than 4%, more than eight words out of 200, more than basically one line or two. You might have to go over it five or six or seven times before you can remember the paragraph. How many senses in a paragraph? About four. Now, out of what it is going to be like maybe 25 different paragraphs. You can remember four and you had to go over this five or six times. What's 25 divided by five? It's five. It's about 5%.

It's right around that 4% mark. So this is one of the human flaws that are built into the brain. Now, the second flaw is that the brain is constantly chattering in the background, the Zen philosophy. We call this the wild monkey, the wild horse, you know, the chattering monkey, all these different types of phrases we have for because the human mind never shuts up. And it's always talking about old stuff. If you listen to your brain, it's going to talk in a stream of consciousness. It never shuts up. It's usually like 90% negative. It's all old information. It's not bringing anything new to the table. It may seem a little new because it's molding it into different shapes and versions of the same old crap, but it's just the same old rubbish. It's junk. That's a defect of the human mind. People worry, get nervous, feel bad, and feel guilty. These are all things that are built into the human brain, literally hardwired this way, programmed this way, and it's not your fault.

So that's what I want to tell you. It's not your fault. You're not alone. Here's between you and everybody else. I'm teaching you specific tool strategies and techniques so you can get out of this Very shortly. I'm going to be doing a Book I think I might title Path to Enlightenment or the University of Life, one of those two. And it's going to be all about enlightenment, how to get out of these traps of mind and have a nice, clear, organized mind that you can actually use to eliminate these built in flaws. Now, those are just your mental defects. A lot of other defects are built in because of your programming. When you were a child, because of traumas that happened during childhood, because of bad inputs into your brain, your brain's a computer. If you get this data, it has these inputs. If it has these experiences, it reacts a certain way. Again, not your fault and you're not alone.

NLP - Visualization - Mind/Body - Sleep

Now here's another great technology you can use. It's called N L P stands for Neuro Linguistic Programming neuro means brain linguistic means language in PE Of course means programming. Now Bandler and Grayndler originally came out with this but Anthony Robbins kind of became the poster child for he's the one that really popularized it and he popularized it in a book called Unlimited Power talked all about neuro linguistic programming. Now I'm showing you a couple of his programs here that I absolutely love. One's called a week in the giant within so much better than the unlimited power book. I absolutely loved it. He only read one book in your life. You should absolutely get that one.

It's got tons of tool strategies and techniques to make your life better and to help understand why your mind works. Now the personal power he had personal power wanted personal power too. I've listened to each one of those programs bit by bit by bit and I can't tell you what the difference is. So if you can pick those up very cheaply online and I'm sure you can find them very cheaply you'll get him either C.D. or DVD form. You might be able to download them on line just different ways to do it but grab that package. Absolutely fantastic. But I want to tell you a little bit about neuro linguistic programming. It's the science of how you change your mind.

So it works in two different ways. One is the science of duplicating success by taking specific talents, specific abilities that people have, analyzing their mindset, how they think about how they picture it, how they hold their body, all these different components and figuring out how you can very rapidly duplicate their success so you can get talents and abilities. They're probably about 80 to 90 percent as good as they have but you can do it in hours, days or weeks instead of months, years and decades. It's so much faster it's absolutely fantastic. But what I want to show you in this program is also the science of how to change your state, how to do a state change, and how to use things like scrambling techniques to help knock down the real emotional content of traumas.

It works absolutely fantastic. So an LP in EMR. Those are the kind of the two therapies that work the best for dealing with old past traumas, for helping you see them as farther away, as distant as light or to literally reprogram the way your brain processes the trauma. Now I can also use it for positive state changes to scientifically figure out how you can achieve the states that you want. So an LP is absolutely fascinating. Some people use this as a standalone therapy. I use it as just a portion of what I do in my therapy programs in my coaching chapters. Absolutely fantastic. If you're really excited about it and you want to learn a little bit more, one of the things that I can do is help you out. I've got an annual PE Book so you can look that up.

Just look at an LP and it'll pop right up. So shameless plug there. Go ahead and grab that you can get that very inexpensively. I'm not charging a lot for that Book. Why I want to get out there to help the masses. So let me ask you a question. Do you know how to duplicate success? If you don't then an LP is the absolute best solution. It's going to show you how to take the qualities, the traits, the thought systems, everything that helps somebody mentally become successful and help you duplicate that. Remember the best way to duplicate success is not to create a new way of doing it. Not to reinvent the wheel but to simply duplicate what's working. I always found this fascinating when you think in your mind the specific words that you use will actually have different emotional impacts.

So if you change your language you literally change your emotions. Sometimes we call this your explanatory style of how you explain things to yourself. That's one way they use language to change feelings. If you describe something as a disaster instead of a challenge obviously you're going to field two different ways. If you see something as a horrific tragedy versus this too shall pass. Those are two different ways of stating the exact same thing but they have wildly different variations in how you feel about it. You know they said that while the Chinese symbol for problem is also the Chinese symbol for opportunity, some languages can be very very powerful.

They talk a lot about neuro linguistic programming because that's how you change your mind through the language that you use and the programs that you create. So language is very powerful. It literally determines how you feel because remember the process you have a thought process which is composed of a bunch of languages that determines how you feel and based on how you feel you take a certain action. So that's how the human mind works. So we want to get this solved upfront at the point of thought in the specific words that we're using. Now the other way you can program the mind because they say a picture is worth what a thousand words. So visualization is very powerful so you always want to picture what you want and not what you don't want. Now you do this with pictures and you also do with language.

Don't say I don't want to worry I don't want to worry I don't want to worry you say I want serenity and don't picture the bad situation going on. Picture the situation you want going on, relaxing by the beach, not getting audited by the IRS, so by reprogramming the mind we change the emotions. The best way to do that is visualization. Now visualization will also activate that small mechanism called the articular activator that shoved up inside underneath the folds of your brain so it's on the bottom center of your brain and what it does is based on what you tell yourself especially what you picture vividly and especially vividly with emotion it will look out into the universe and it will scan the environment to find things to help you accomplish that. So if you're going to get a new car all of a sudden you'll see every magazine and television ad newspaper and anybody talking about cars going by billboards that say hey come on down.

We've got a great deal. We've got zero percent interest whatever you're focusing on. The particular activator will kick in because you're visualizing it and help you to get your goal. Now unfortunately as you can see my wife's thinking about diamonds is a problem. I've got to get her to picture other things so visualization is very powerful and you'll see amazing results now with visualization is not only about getting what you want. It's about changing your state. Think of it this way when you worry you picture certain things when you get depressed you picture certain things. When you have low self-esteem you picture certain things when you're phobic you picture certain things the people that don't have these challenges versus the people that do have wildly different visualization patterns.

They picture different things. I used to go to the office every day and picture all the bad things that could happen. The winners and the achievers were picturing all the great things that could happen, all the great things that they could accomplish. I was doing the formula right. But in the wrong direction so don't picture what you don't want. Now this isn't a delusion. This isn't kidding yourself. It's just keeping your brain in your particular activator focused on what you do want instead of what you don't want. It'll help you get more of what you want and it'll give you a much more positive state. Believe me, focusing on and visualizing those negative things that are actually the least likely to happen is more delusional than picturing positive things that may or may not happen. Makes sense.

Now let's talk a little bit about the mind-body connection. These two systems are totally interactive. They're getting so interactive it's getting hard to figure out where one starts and the other one stops. So two different strategies that you can use. One is to change your body and that will actually have an impact on and change your mind. We talked about diet. We talked about exercise do these things in a positive direction and you'll not only see changes in your body but you'll gain new neurotransmitters stress logo down muscular tension will go down the body impacts the mind now as significantly probably even more significantly if you change your mind you're going to change your body your mind is constantly sending out signals.

When you have a thought when you have a feeling it interacts with every single cell in the body and the transfer of that information is virtually instantaneous. It's amazingly fast. It creates changes in immune system and digestion and blood flow and neurotransmitters and endocrine systems and bile and muscular tension and on and on and on and on and on all the way through every single cell every single system. That's why positive thinking is so important. It's programming not just your mind but also impacting your body.

This is why positive relationships are so important because if you have that negativity going through your mind of a negative relationship it's also going through your body and damaging every single system. So they're even finding that your mind is not necessarily your brain, just your brain between your ears. There's intelligence in every cell of the body: a blood cell can produce another blood cell with no signal from the brain. It simply does it on its own. There's also neuro tissue which is all your brain is made of. It's a clump of neural tissue. They find these clumps of neural tissue throughout your body.

So like little tiny brains they're finding this in your heart, in your stomach, in your digestive tract and your muscles. So the brain works more like the Internet where the the brain itself is the central hub but there's all these sub computers these sub hubs these sub pieces that are talking to each other. So the brain or mind directs everything but it's not just in one central location. It's carried throughout the body. Absolutely fascinating. So take care of the mind and your body is going to function better. Take care of your body and your mind is going to function better now every problem you've ever had. I want you to know that somebody has already had it. They've already found a solution and they've already beat it.

So where can you find these things? The first place that I started was the library. Somebody had written it down somewhere in this day and age. I use YouTube a lot and Google a lot. I go to the blogs a lot. I'll even ask for recommendations on places like linked it and say if it's a professional question you can go to read it if it's a non-professional question you can pore through the search engine. You can look through the research journals. Somebody somewhere you've got the largest store of information ever held by a human being right in your computer. Make sure you get really good at researching and finding things and going out there and pooling the resources that you like to use.

So don't try to solve your problem simply by thinking in your head. My gosh , how can I solve this if I have to spend more than five to 15 minutes figuring out my head. I'm already going to a resource. It's faster, it's better and they'll come up with thoughts and ideas and solutions that I never even would have ever come up with. Never would have thought that it might take me to another branch of thought or another way to solve my challenge and get me looking at new and exciting areas. So a lot of times even if I can come up with the answer I don't want to because I'll come up with one answer.

But by researching on the internet I might come up with a half dozen different answers: better ways of doing things or better ways of doing things in a certain situation or at a certain time in life or with certain people or a way to take this one solution and extrapolate it to other areas of my life. So I leave you with this thought every problem here that somebody has already had. They've already beaten it and they've already told you how to fix it. That's amazingly empowering now a quick word about addiction. When I was doing mental health therapy they used to have a phrase they said addiction is primary. What does it mean? It means it's number one.

Nothing is ever gonna get better until the addiction is beat. I don't care if you have 20 different diagnosis you're ADHD and you're autistic and you've got bipolar and you're depressed and you've got anxiety. Doesn't matter what you have until we get you clean and sober we can't begin to work on any of those other things. So addiction is always the number one thing to be. And then once you've beaten that it makes it so much easier to beat everything out. So if you're having any challenges, any problems with addiction or a person in your life is having problems or challenges with addiction. Here's what I'll tell you. AA and any Alcoholics Anonymous and Narcotics Anonymous tend to work the best.

They give good group support. Here's the recovery rate to go to a therapist. The recovery rates are 26 percent for an AA or any meeting. It's 25 percent. There's only a 1 percent difference. And I'm not telling you that AA is superior to therapy. Not necessarily. I had 90 percent success rates. ACE didn't change. Why? Because I brought in coping skills I brought in the A and A I brought in different therapy techniques I brought in multiple coping skills I brought in social workers and psychiatrists and medication and all these different things employment that AA couldn't touch. That's how I got really high. Ninety percent success rate. So the best package is to have therapy and AA. Now that increases and multiplies the effect of either.

So I think it's best to have both. But if you're broke you just want to put a big toe in the water. You're not sure what to do to get to an AA meeting. Get to the end of a meeting AA is Alcoholics Anonymous but don't let the name fool you. If that's the only meeting in the area and say you're doing cocaine you're like Oh I'm not an alcoholic. I can't go to that because I'm tired out in the studio audience. 90 percent of people in that room do alcohol and another substance if you go to an AA meeting 90 percent of those people do substances but also 90 percent also do alcohol. So there's so much overlap in the 12 steps that they're doing are virtually identical.

So it doesn't matter. I mean if I weren't there in the first five minutes of an A or an AA meeting I couldn't tell the difference between the two because they announced at the beginning of the meeting and then just kind of done then they all at the same start work on the 12 steps and they start reading from their books and they start sharing their experience strength and hope maybe there's a Q and A you know it's all support from the group and it works fantastic. Now if you have a problem with addiction but the problem is you are living with somebody with addiction or you're somebody that has an addiction that you love, get to Al Anon Al Anon is short for Alcoholics Anonymous. It's a family based program for the people that are affected by addiction.

So you can learn what to do to help them and what not to do to help them how addiction works and if you can deal with some of your issues if you've been around somebody who's an addict for a long period of time they probably seriously impacted you. So in every way shape and form of your family member or friend, some of it's close to an addict, Al Anon will help you. Alan is the one that came up with the phrase give us six chapters and if you're not satisfied I will gladly refund your misery.

So the recommendation is always go to six hour nine meetings or go to six AA meetings try it out give it a chance you probably can be very satisfied very rare that if you're six meaning somebody is not happy with al anon or AA don't go once because your brain is going to say oh I don't want this I don't need this is gonna be searching for every way that this doesn't apply to you by the sixth meeting you'll definitely know how it applies to you you'll have gained some new skills you'll have gotten some support from the group and you'll realize yes this program can help me here's the other critical key to feeling great.

You need to get good sleep. Sleep is fundamental. It's like a diet. It's like exercise but a lot of people don't think about it. Now who are the people that don't think about it? The people that are actually getting enough but not quite enough. If you've got insomnia. Believe me you think about it. And if you've got insomnia you've got to get some treatment for that. Now some simple things you can do to get better sleep are adjusting the role. What do I mean by that? Not too hot, not too cold. If anything it should be a little bit cooler. People tend to sleep better just like this lady. Here you have a little bit of blanket over you but you want to stick your arms or your legs out.

You probably want to be like her. I'll be wearing a bra to bed. Don't be wearing anything constricting some loose underwear or a nightgown or some loose pajamas. It's best to have the skin exposed. So this might be the perfect outfit for a lady. GUY MIGHT JUST BE THERE IN HIS UNDERWEAR. That allows your skin to breathe. If you become dehydrated or too hot or too cold these things are going to wake you up. So the right temperature level on the cool side is enough so you can have a sheet or a blanket over you that creates comfort and also creates the appropriate amount of warmth. Now the room can't have any noise and the alarm clock wakes you up so noise wakes people up and disturbs sleep. By definition so you don't have any background noise if you can avoid it.

Now some people like relaxation music in the background. Some people sleep with the TV on or they play a little music. I understand that. But you know what traffic noise is. You don't want things that are clunking. You don't want to hear you know the radiator pounding these types of things. Keep it as peaceful as possible. Now the first thing that triggers the sleep process is you closing your eyes when it gets dark. That's when you release melatonin. So melatonin you can take is a supplement that's certainly helpful. It also helps with sleep cycles. It's a naturally occurring hormone. Just don't overdo it. I would take one milligram or half a milligram and increase it from there and don't go over the three milligrams.

OK read the bottle. Now when you close your eyes when it's dark the melatonin is released and you start to go to sleep but as little as 1 loom. That's one candle light ten feet away. That's how strong one loom is. This is going to disturb your sleep. Do you like to see one low from about a mile away? If it's not foggy that's how strong that is. So your eyes are very sensitive to light so you want to pitch dark. You should barely be able to see your hand in front of your face and it's better if you can't see your hand in front of your face. A little bit of light can really disturb your sleep. So right temperature, no light , no sound if you can avoid it or some relaxing sounds that help you to sleep and you want to make sure that you're not dehydrated.

I've been having trouble sleeping lately because I live in Florida. The A.C. runs all the time. It dehydrates the air it condensates and goes out through the AC system so it's amazingly dry. So if I don't have a little humidifier by the bed I will dehydrate. My mouth will almost dry up and I'll get so thirsty I have to get up in the middle of the night so have a little bit of water before you go to sleep so you don't get dehydrated but not enough that it wakes you up because you have to go to the bathroom. They used to call that the inland Indian alarm clock. When the Native Americans wanted to have somebody wake them up in the morning they would pick one of the Indians and they would drink a bunch of water. In about six to eight hours they'd have to get up to pee.

Whereas all the other Indians might be sleeping and you know eight nine ten eleven twelve hours. So that was the Indian alarm clock. Make sure you're not doing that. So not too much water so that you wake up in not too little so that you get dehydrated and wake up. You want the perfect balance. So those are all your good sleep. KEYES for now. Oh one more. Go ahead. If you have anything that you're worrying about or anything that you're thinking about, write it down on a piece of paper and leave it on the counter. A lot of times these thoughts will loop through your head because you worry that you're going to forget him or you're not going to dress the next day. This is a great technique to help you sleep better. And you want to try to keep approximately the same sleep pattern.

Go to bed at the same time and get up at the same time. Now before I wrap up this chapter I want to tell you something that's amazingly important: nobody is coming to the rescue. I have to tell people they are in therapy, you know. I'm your therapist. I'm about the only person that's ever coming to the rescue but I'm not going to go home and I'm not going to fix your problems. You got to go home and you got to fix your problems. I give you tool strategy techniques but you gotta do it. So unlike when you're a little kid you can't just fail and your parents will come and they'll pick you up and society will pick you up and the school will pick you up and you know all these people friends and relatives will come and pick you up.

I'm telling you nobody's coming to the rescue so failure is not an option. So get out there and kick some butt. They say if it's going to be it's up to me. That's absolutely true. Make it happen and here's your second tip. Don't be a victim. Why? Because victims don't get better. OK. I'm not a rape victim. I'm a rape survivor. OK. I'm not an alcoholic. I'm a grateful recovering alcoholic. Alcoholics drink but a grateful recovering alcoholic recovering alcoholics don't drink. And if you're grateful all the better. Right. So be very careful about the words that you use in the way that you picture yourself. Now I'm also saying don't be a victim in terms of oh poor me poor me poor me.

You know what was me and whining—complaining playing the victim role. You'll never ever get any better. And when you whine—complain here's what's happening out there in the audience. Fifty percent of people don't care and the other half are glad it's you. Don't whine [REMOVED] and complain. You could only solve a problem by solving a problem. That's fine to ask for help but nobody is going to do it for you. It's up to you. And I know I absolutely know you can do it. You've survived everything up to now and ask for help. Get out there, get the tools, get the resources. You've made a great step by getting this program. There's so much more help to be had out there if you need additional help.

Please go and get it. I've never had anybody that came to me for help and say boy I as I look back I wish I waited longer. Now they all say to the man woman or child I wish I got here earlier how earlier, usually years and years and years earlier, they knew the help was there but they just sat day after day literally sitting in their crap waiting for things to mysteriously get better. They don't mysteriously get better, they get better when you take action. That's your final tip for now and I'll see you in the very next chapter.

Perfectionism - Maladaptive Behaviors - Reality Therapy

Now let me teach you a little bit about perfectionism. I consider perfectionism a mental illness. Now it's not in the DSM the Diagnostic and Statistical Manual but I have it penciled in mind. It's a form of neurosis neurosis is when you think a certain thought or a certain belief system member that stands for B.S. to remind you what it is that hurts you. So working against you is neurotic thinking perfectionism is neurotic thinking since telling you some very important perfection does not exist. So when you try to do things perfectly you don't get things done. And perfectionism is just a way for you to make you feel bad about yourself because you can't be perfect and hello nothing in the universe is perfect everything. If you drill down you'll find it in perfection.

So use this philosophy instead believe that good enough is good enough. I remember I was taught this term in management class. They said hey what would you rather do? Would you rather create one item that's perfect that sells for ten dollars or would you rather make five of these that are good enough. The customers were thrilled with him. They're not exactly perfect but they're 98 percent perfect. Great. One person is gonna make 10 dollars and one person is gonna make 50. Would you rather be the person with the one perfect item that sold or the five almost perfect items that sold? You want to be the guy that's making five times as much. So good enough literally is good enough. Drive on.

I just want you to hold in your mind that perfectionism is a mental illness. Walk away from it. Perfection does not exist. So eliminate this thought system. This belief within your mind. Be creative and think of as many ways as possible to knock it down in your own mind. You'll start to come up with new systems. Why perfectionism is crazy. Let it go. Now it's very important to be happy. Why? Because this is a scientific fact. Later doesn't exist, the past doesn't exist. The future doesn't exist only that now exists. You need to be happy now. We talked to one of the earlier chapters about happily achieving. That's very important so even when you're doing work tasks and things that aren't that pleasant.

Figure out how you can make them a little bit fun. Make them a little bit pleasant and enjoy them. Now don't say I will take a vacation next year or the year after the year after. Go out and take one now if it's been a while take one now I can remember when I went for five six seven years without ever taking a vacation cause I just wanted to get everything done I was slamming and slamming is slamming. I tell you I was a human being. I was not a human being. I was not really enjoying my life at the fullest level. I made the mistake that I'm telling you not to be happy now when people are trying to be happy later doesn't really exist. So go ahead and enjoy yourself now. Have fun now.

Get out there now weather reasons later doesn't exist either is it's actually a mental trick one of the things that I used to do is when people used to procrastinate I would say Hey don't tell yourself you're not going to procrastinate because your brain knows you procrastinate all the time it's gonna go B.S. It's not going to believe you and that affirmation isn't going to work. Here's what I want you to do I want you to work really hard now and tell your brain not I'm not going to procrastinate I'm going to procrastinate Absolutely and I procrastinate but I'm going to do it tomorrow I'm going to procrastinate Tomorrow well tomorrow just like later doesn't exist because you're always in today so tomorrow what do you tell yourself.

Oh it's not that I'm going to procrastinate I'm absolutely going to procrastinate but I'm going to do it tomorrow and then the next day and the next day and the next day play the same trick. It's a great mental trick. This is how you use the trick for yourself instead of against yourself, so be happy now if your brain wants you to be sad. Now say you know what. Absolutely I'm going to be sad but it's going to be tomorrow and then the play the same game again tomorrow so get out there enjoy your life your life your purpose in life are only a few things to enjoy and suck the joy out of every single moment to learn grow and become more and to share these great gifts of happiness learning enjoy with others that's literally the purpose of life and if you miss out on being happy I don't think any of the other ones actually matter here that again if you're not happy I don't think any of those other ones actually matter least they won't help you so be happy now.

Now here's the second part of that. Stop seeking happiness outside of yourself and I'm gonna give you one simple reason because it doesn't exist outside of yourself. Happiness like every other mental state happens within you. Now sometimes there's certain things like somebody hands you a million dollars in something outside of your triggers and you say oh if I ever get a million dollars then I'll be happy. That's simply happiness happening inside of you with an outside stimulus. But you don't need that outside stimulus to feel happy. You can simply enjoy everything around you. You can enjoy the peace and serenity of the moment. You can go through a final memory of feeling good but all happiness happens inside. This is why depressed people aren't happy because no matter what happens on the outside because they're not happy on the inside they refuse to trigger it almost regardless of what happens on the outside.

They can't be happy. They're not triggered by those outside things to create that internal happiness that's what depression is. Somebody hands a depressed person a million dollars and they say great. Now I've got to pay taxes on it. Great. Now somebody's trying to come by and steal it. Great. Why did I get this 20 years ago when I was young enough to enjoy it when I really needed it. Great. Just put it on the counter. They're just not stimulated by it so don't seek happiness outside yourself seek it within yourself this technique. This strategy is absolutely key. Here's a way to break free of old maladaptive behaviors simply by asking one question. This is an old Dr. Phil favorite set.

How's that working for you? You know we do this in reality therapy all the time. We use the phrase "how's that working for you?" And if somebody says Hey that does not work and great for me because obviously that's why they're in therapy right. It's not working great. Take that maladaptive behavior and get rid of it. I tell people I say well how's that working for you. They say it's horrible. I say how long you've been trying to work it that way. And they say oh I don't know five 10 15 20 40 years. I go OK you know 20 to 40 years is probably long enough to work a failed experiment. Why don't we try something different? See how I don't I don't just say let's try something different. I have to get them to get rid of the old behavior.

So what I do is I let him see how futile it is by saying 10 to 20 years is long enough to work a failed experiment that helps them to drop the old behavior. Then they and I sit down and we look at how you would like to think and how you would like to look at things. How would you like to do things in such a way that it actually works for you. And how about if we can make it fast, simple and easy. And even if it's not truly fast, simple and easy it's gonna be faster, simpler and easier than the old maladaptive behavior. And they're going to get much better results. So I tell him hey if you can survive things getting worse and worse. If you could survive for 10 to 20 years we're going to have this failed system. Could you give it two weeks for the new system to work see how I line that up.

Perfect. So look at your old maladaptive behaviors and ask yourself a simple question. How's that working for you? Is this really the way I want my life to be? Am I willing to keep acting the same way and getting the same results or do I want to try something different. When would now be a good time to change now. Now we talked a little bit about reality therapy and I got the quote here: reality is a fine concept. You know that's kind of what I always say to clients. You know what a concept to actually be based in reality. Isn't that mind blowing. Why is it mind blowing? Because so few people are based in reality. They're mostly based on their illusions and delusions. OK so they rarely step in reality. Look at the last person we just talked about.

They've been working on a failed plan for 10 20 30 40 years. Is that reality based? No, that's not reality based delusional erroneous thinking thinking that is an error. So let's try reality for a little while. So the first part of reality therapy is how's that working for you if you don't like it then let's look at the reality of the situation. Say you're in a bad relationship. This relationship has been bad for five 10-15 years. Guess what. If nothing changes physics 1 or 1 says an object in motion tends to remain in motion unless acted upon. Which means if we're gonna do the same thing that we did before we're gonna keep getting the same results. They say if you always do what you always did you'll always get what you always got. Definition of insanity doing the same thing over and over again expecting different results. These are all ways to describe using reality therapy. There are some therapists.

Reality therapy is all they use. If you've ever readed an episode of Dr. Phil this is about 90 percent of what he uses. He'll sneak in a couple other therapy styles that are helpful or he doesn't even realize he's blending in. But basically he is doing reality therapy. Does this make sense when you look at it from outside reality based truth time? No lies, no delusions. Take away all those delusions, illusions , get rid of them. Here's what the situation really is. Once you clearly see a situation then the solution becomes obvious. You've been in a bad relationship for five or 10 years. You've tried everything, it's never gonna get any better. What do you think the chances are the next five or 10 years are going to look about the same in the personal sayings?

Pretty close to a hundred percent you go. That's exactly right. Do you want to spend another five or 10 years of the only life you ever get 5 or 10 of the best years of your life. Do you want to give them up simply to be in the same pain that you came and you told me originally the answer is No. This is how to take people and illusions. Look at their problems objectively without the illusion and then when they actually see it in their mind they can twist it in front of somebody else who refuses to accept any answer except the reality based answer. The delusions dissolve. How can you dissolve the illusions you have in your mind? I sometimes describe my therapy as disillusioning people and people are like disillusioned that that sounds kind of negative.

Isn't it funny that we think of disillusionment as a negative term? Listen to the word dis illusion. This means to remove and then there's illusion. I'm removing your illusions and somehow you see that as a negative. Most people when they come to a therapist if they're delusional either take medication or they go into therapy with somebody like me and you remove the illusions. They pay you good money to do that. So why is disillusionment a negative concept? I'm telling you it's not your illusions that are causing you your pain. And when you can see past your own illusions you get back to reality. You don't need me anymore as a therapist. You can solve it. So get real objective about your problems.

Look at them from the outside. Maybe use somebody else as a sounding board. Maybe go to therapy whatever you need to do to see things clearly. And then the solution will simply float to the top. I love this one. This is a quote from the big book that says acceptance is the answer to all my problems today. We have to look through our lives and say who are what are you refusing to accept the pain you have in your life the ongoing pain that you have in your life usually is a resistance to reality because the reality is maybe of a negative person in your life but it's who keeps them in your life you but you're refusing to accept that.

So whatever you refuse to accept, whatever you hide from yourself, whatever you cover an illusion or delusions right, you are going to keep there's some things that you refuse to accept that are also true. You say well I've got a crappy boss who wanted two things. Except that you have a crappy boss OK. And get over it. That removes the pain. Simply accept it. Hey there, crappy. So stop talking about stop worrying about spending any time thinking about it because they're going to be the same about 20 years from now. So get over it by accepting it or accept the fact that you have a crappy boss and realize you know there's thousands of other positions in your field that you would not be within the same company as this person. You can simply quit and go work for somebody else.

I used to either do that if I had a really negative boss or here's what else I would do. I would go to school with them. I found that they were working for me. Then we had a totally different relationship. Isn't that funny. So I would get a master's degree. I would leapfrog over them and then they would be working for me and all of a sudden they were sweet as pie or in the worst case scenario. They weren't sweet as pie. They really were a complete jerk. It was totally outside their control. But now I could fire them but you can't just sit there not accepting something that is called frustration. One of the reasons you get so frustrated in life is a signal. It's a signal that there's something you could be doing in your life but you're not doing it and therefore it's painful. It's a pain signal. So what's going on in your life?

What situation are you refusing to accept in your life that you could be solving but you're not solving. See how that works. So look at who or what you're refusing to accept then accept it and then make the necessary changes and you will do absolutely fantastic now to wrap up this chapter. I want to share with you a wonderful mystical place. It's called and it's a magical place where no negativity exists. You know why. Because I banish everything that's negative from my life. If there's negative people around me I get rid of them. Doesn't matter if they're family members, I get rid of them. My sister was being really negative one Thanksgiving and I threw her out of the house. I haven't seen her since. Some people say oh you can't get rhythm, they're family. Now sometimes families are the perfect people to get rid of.

So I don't have any negative friends in my life. I don't have any negative co-workers in my life. I don't have any negative significant others in my life. My wife is beautiful, kind and loving. I specifically picked her because she really didn't have a negative bone in her body. Perfect. I don't live in a crappy home environment. I have a nice home. Even when I lived in a very cheap place I made sure it was in a nice neighborhood. It was cheap because you know I was going to school and I didn't have much money and I would rent from individuals as opposed to go to an apartment complex because you know there wouldn't be a lot of other poor people around me and these types of things are you know gangs and drug dealers and you know living in the crack hole and these types of things.

So I had a very small place but I kept it very nice. I kept it as a positive environment. You can do other things to make it a positive environment. I don't live in a crime district so although the crime rates may be such and such a statistic there about one tenth of that where I live. Why? Because I live in Portland. I made sure of these things. There may be a lot of unemployment out there in the world but I got four different degrees. Why? Because that way I would always be employed or over employed. I sometimes have a second or third job gone. I can't get to all the work I want to do. So this doesn't happen unemployment doesn't happen in Portland. Why? Because I set it up that way. So always remove all forms and negativity and there's a lot of different forms that we talked about. We talked about negative things about France.

We talked about negative and significant ideas. We talked about negative family members. We talked about negative environments, we talked about crime. We talked about employment. So there's all these things that you can help to remove at least in the nineteen ninety five percentile out of your land and create a beautiful land like land where no negativity exists. Make that happen. The environment that you're in is huge; it's either supporting you or dragging you down. Think about that. Hear that again. You see they're supporting you or dragging you down. It's worth doing whatever you need to do to create this kind of environment. I want you to have that kind of environment. You deserve that kind of environment: your family, your loved ones, your significant other deserves that kind of environment. Go out there. Make it happen.

Fear - Illusion Of Weakness - Reframing

Now let's discuss the issue of fear. A lot of people are having challenges with this and they don't even know it. Think about it this way. Anxiety and depression are both fear based. Did you realize that anxiety means you're afraid of the future? You're worried something's going to happen in the future. We call it worry But worry is a very cute way of saying fear. Depression is the same thing. It's fear that things are never ever ever going to get better. They're both fear based. So we have to let go of the fear. Fear is also known as false evidence appearing real. We don't know for sure that bad things are going to happen in the future.

Matter of fact if you tested yourself and everything you ever worried that would happen in the future that was bad pretty much less than 1 percent of it ever happened. And whether you worried about it or not you would have dealt with it. About 90 percent as well had never worried about it. If you spent years worrying about it, you would notice that only one percent of everything you ever worry about actually happens. The other 9 9 percent is a waste and it's destroying your life. That's reason enough to let it go. And even for that one percent rarely if ever all but you can count on one hand all of the things that you worried about that actually helped you when the thing occurred. It's exceedingly rare.

It's like one thing in one hundred or one thing in a thousand closer to one thing in a thousand. Right. Same thing with depression. You're worried that things will never get better. There's a famous quote that says we have nothing to fear but fear itself. Your depression is what's causing things to never get better. It's a Catch 22. Things would get better if you weren't so—depressed. You're so—depressed. Things can't get any better. So what you have to do is get rid of the Depression. We've shown you tons of different ways you can do it here. If you're still having challenges with anxiety and depression, remember to go out and get some extra help.

There's support groups. There's therapy, there's medication, there are all the different strategies that we talked about here. There's self-help books that help get on top of the anxiety and get on top of the Depression now knowing that fear is one way that you can get out of it. Why? Because you know that most of the fears aren't real. So you're free to let them go and to get better. You need to let them go. Now having said that I want to talk to you about the illusion of weakness. You are actually amazingly powerful. Think about it regardless of what's happened in your life, how bad it's been. All the horrific things that have happened I want you to know something.

You have survived every single challenge ever thrown at you and there might have been a little bit of damage done there's some hurt that's done. That happens to everybody. But you survived it and you can survive much more. Some of you are much stronger than I am. How do I know that because you survived more and those things that don't break us tend to make us stronger. So some of you actually have gotten stronger from all the challenges. You're simply tired. It's been a marathon, it's been a long run. You can deal with this stuff for a long time. You're simply tired. You need to rest up being tired after a marathon doesn't mean you're weak. The guy that runs I think it's what 24 to 26 miles they run the Boston Marathon. The guy who wins.

He's feeling very weak. Why? Because he's tired it doesn't make him a loser. Hello. He won the Boston Marathon. He is the strongest person there but you'd probably see him rolling around on the ground because he can't even stand up anymore. So at that point he looks at himself and says My God I'm weak and he's not wrong but he's not really weak. His body in his mind simply needs a little bit of time to recover. I think you're a lot like that. You just need a little bit of time to recover and you need to stop creating the damage. We've talked about a lot of the different ways that we hurt ourselves. There's an old expression that says out of all the people that have hurt me in life. I'm the person that hurt me the most.

So when you stop hurting you then you can give yourself a good rest. Let some of this stuff in the past go relax, refresh , rejuvenate. We've shown you some of the ways to do that. I just want you to know that your weakness is literally a piece of fiction. You are one of the strongest people that are out there now. Your next great strategy is to increase your response ability. Look at how many different ways you can respond to a given situation. I remember when I first started doing therapy they said if a client ever has a situation ever has a problem ever asked a question ever needs help in a certain way and you don't know the answer.

Here's what you need to do before you come in the next day. You have to figure out three ways to respond to that client to give them those solutions. You can have more but three is the minimum. So in any area of your life you need to start doing this as a research project. You say well I don't know how to deal with how to start a conversation in a social situation. I don't know how to deal with it when somebody says something negative about me. I don't know how to say something to somebody when I know I should. I don't know how to be assertive and then figure out at least three ways that you can solve those things. Simple trip over to YouTube will solve those things.

I'll bet you could go back to this Book and find at least two or three ways to solve each one of your challenges. Just go back through the Book and look for that specific one. Ask some friends to read some self-help books. There's resources out there that will help you increase your responsibility and your ability to respond. This is your job in life. Human beings are creatures of adaptation which means we can adapt to any situation. Now instead of reinventing the wheel it's best to find the specific tools and strategies like the ones that I'm teaching you here that can simply be handed to you. So a Book of self-help book therapy is a real legitimate shortcut.

These are all great resources to increase your responsibility. You can even become a responsible fan. I guess I would call it somebody who is a connoisseur of finding response abilities for situations that haven't even come up yet say you've never been given a major award. But how would you handle it if you were maybe not married yet. How would you handle things at your wedding? How would you handle asking somebody to be your bridesmaid or your best man. Start gaining all these coping skills. I'm a therapist so whenever I find a new coping skill whether I've ever had a client that needed it whether I need it or not I grab it. I'm just a collector of these things.

So start collecting coping skills and you'll either use them for yourself or you'll use them for somebody else this technique I love. It's called The Power of reframing. Reframing is literally like putting a new frame around an old picture. It makes it look totally different. So also known as spin spin doctors go out there for politicians and one guy says well this guy stole a million dollars from the American people his spin doctor comes in and says no. I put that money aside for you. I reallocated it over here. Aren't you lucky that I did that for you? You're welcome. So that's reframing. How can I look at something in such a way that it's positive versus negative that it helps me versus hurting me. Now I've got to be very careful of the power of reframing when you're anxious.

It takes things that are positive or that are neutral or maybe mildly negative and makes them wildly negative. It reframes them in such a way that it makes it worse instead of better. Depression takes something that's mildly negative or neutral or sometimes even positive and makes it into a negative. It reframes it. That's why anxiety and depression seem so real because your reframes have a certain logic to them that if you buy into them you say oh my god yes that's horrible. And that's so true. But you have to realize when you're reading politicians spin things you realize that there's an infinite number of ways to spin things. You should be spinning things, reframing things to work for you not against you to help you feel better, not worse to give you the energy you need to beat the problem instead of draining it out of you.

So you can't reframing is absolutely huge. When I first started doing therapy they said if you can't do anything but reframe things that was your only therapy style you would be a great therapist. So getting really good at reframing this will help you see things better. Help you do better in life and you can reframe things for other people. This helps them feel better. And by reframing things they won't know that you're quite unquote doing therapy with them or trying to alter the way that they see things. You'll just do a gentle refrain. It'll chapter through like butter. They'll never even really know you did it. If you're subtle about it and it will create a state change for them they'll feel better, more empowered, more resourceful and you'll have done that wonderful, now different kind of refrain.

I call this the effective use of lying to yourself. People look at life as a negative thing, not necessarily a lot of people lie to themselves. They do those negative reframes, those negative re frames are absolutely lies in life 98 percent of the time they're lies but they're very effective in changing your state and changing what you'll do or won't do. If you can be effective or not be effective. I use a little joke here. I'm not actually a doctor but I play one on TV. Go ahead and bend over we're going to give you this shot right now so a funny way of looking at it but they say it's fake until you make it. That's one effective use of lying to yourself. Even though you're not a recovering addict yet because you know you're barely sober, maybe as sober for a day.

But just imagine doing the things that somebody had been sober for two years would do. They would go to meetings, they would talk to their sponsor and they sure as hell wouldn't drink or drug perfectly. So you kid yourself you fake it until you make it you lie to yourself until you get there. I used to do this in college. College was going to be long, painful , boring , expensive and it was going to tire the heck out of me because I really hardly got any sleep for about two years. But what I did was I used the effective use of lying to myself. I said this won't last long. This will be fun. I'm just going to eat pizza and talk to my buddies and read the pretty girls go by sitting in an air conditioned environment.

I'm just looking at pictures and turning the pages clock's going to tick tick tick tick. I don't even have to do anything. And this whole thing's going to go by. That was an effective use of lying to myself in an effective use of reframing myself. Now the strange thing is if you fake it till you make it, if you use this effective use of lying to yourself by the time you finish lying to yourself it's actually true. When I got up there for graduation for that bachelor's degree another two years had gone by. I finished the second half. I jumped back into college and it seemed like it was just breezing by. I really did just hang out in an air conditioned environment. I did hang out with my buddies. I readed the pretty girls go by and ate a lot of pizza. We didn't slap each other on the back.

You know we went out to nightclubs and had fun and had laughs. We drank too much and laughed too much. We had a good time. There were some good memories. So a lot of what I told myself that I thought was a lie. By the time I finished lying to myself it had become true in my reality. A lot of people who do this say they're trying to start a business to say well I'm going to start a business and they lie to themselves oh this will be easy and I'll just do this and that and boom boom boom boom. Pretty soon on my own business. But then when it takes longer than expected it's harder than expected. They just say Don't worry, it's kind of happening. And when it actually happens they look back and all they have is all that pain, all that struggle all that time just becomes a great part of their story.

The lie becomes true. So great technique given the fact that you're lying to yourself anyways when you get anxiety depression low self-esteem you're telling yourself life's no good I'm no good. You know everything is not good, that's a lie. If you're going to lie, you should at least lie in such a way that it helps you. Given the fact that we're lying anyways that's why this is the effective use of lying to yourself. Exactly. Depression low self-esteem that's the ineffective use of lying yourself. Notice how effective that system is bad. What if you just did the opposite because you're obviously OK with using this system. What if you used it in your favor instead of against yourself. Makes sense. Fantastic. Now here's another great coping mechanism.

I am always shocked at how many people do nothing to it. Hey I was great and if these five things didn't happen to me that I have been double super awesome. That's a real word double super awesome. I'll just raise my kids and I'll make sure these five things don't happen. OK. Then you make five new exciting new mistakes and your kids come out about the same or a little worse than you. Parenting is a major stressor. Here's why. Because of what I just described people do nothing to parenting. They think they can be a parent and there's nothing to it. Think of it this way. What do I have to do to go out and give one piece of advice to a parent? I've got to get a four year degree called the bachelors. I got to get another four year degree.

Call the Masters. I got to do two years of internship reading other people counsel families. I have to go out and get a license that may take me another year. I'm about 10 -11 years into this and I can give a parent one piece of advice. Great but I know a thousand times what they know about parenting. A lot of times parents would look at me and they would say Hey , do you have any kids yourself like that was a great qualifier. And the funny thing is I would have to say to him I've had thousands. Why? Because I've had thousands of patients I understand that you only have three children and they laugh and say "How could you have thousands?" Because that's how many families I've helped. Do I have any personally? No, I have to. I have

guardian and I've helped thousands of people with their children. We have great success rates when people use the tools when they use the skills in every one of those thousand children who have horrible problems. I didn't get to have a nice easy child to deal with and it looks like you haven't either. So let me help you here. And that would move them past this whole concept that you had to be a parent to actually understand parenting. Most parents don't understand parenting. They haven't trained for it and they don't read what other parents are doing. I had the experience of thousands of different families struggling with things. That's more experience than me raising one kid. That's ridiculous. So go out there and learn some parenting skills because nothing can stress you like your kids.

Relationship Skills - ProActive - Journaling

Now this is another key human relationship area that I am absolutely shocked about. Just like parenting , all we do all day long is relate to other people. It's one of our primary functions but so few people have had even one class, one Book, read one book on relationship skills they've never had any personal coaching on. It's not taught in schools and is not taught anywhere you're supposed to kind of pick it up as you go along. Literally the blind leading the blind bad communicators chapter the next generation of bad communicators. So I'm getting slightly better, some getting slightly worse but most of them are horrible at this. They don't know the basic fundamentals of relationship skills but they expect to have good relationships.

And then when they don't have good relationships they blame life. They blame God. They blame themselves, they blame society. Blame a lot of areas most of which have nothing to do with it. So I want you to empower yourself and realize that you don't have to be one of these people whether in therapy or through specific chapters through self-help books you can learn practice and perfecting these relationship skills. Let me give you a couple here just to get you started. So in any relationship we like people that are like us we love people that want to listen to us.

Most people are starving for somebody to listen to. They'll come in, they'll pay me five hundred dollars an hour just to sit there and listen. Now they're thrilled if I give some great advice but the bulk of what they're looking for is simply somebody to actively listen to them. So good listening skills are absolutely huge. People are also starved for appreciation. Rarely does anybody walk up to somebody and say hey it was great when you did this or it was great when you did that or I admire you for this I admire you for that even though they think these things they don't say them out loud one of the worst relationship barriers in child parent relationships is that the parents simply never told their child that they were proud of them. And you ask the parent, are you proud of your child? Go Absolutely. And you go.

When was the last time you told your child and they said oh I I must have done that a dozen times. And then he asked the kids if they would say no. So showing appreciation is huge. Here's how to have a good relationship with anybody: try to be extra nice to them. Notice how nice they are to you and be a little bit nicer to them which you're going to notice is the law. Reciprocity is going to kick in they're going to start being nicer to you. So you try to be even a little nicer than that. This is how me and my wife started having a great relationship. We started to try to outdo each other. I try to be nicer to her and she was to me she tried to be nicer to me than I was to her. And we had this wonderful positive spiral until we really didn't need the technique anymore. We were just constantly trying to think of nice fun little things little touches where we could let the other person know that we love them and we cared about them.

We wanted to be with them and they were important and we let go of all the petty things that weren't worth damaging their relationship for. So learning relationship skills is absolutely a huge help as a few tips get you started. But there's so much more to learn. This could be a 10 hour Book in and of itself. Somebody would say it could be a thousand hour Book but get out there and learn them your life will go significantly better at home at work out there in the environment everywhere the quality of your relationships is going to be the quality of your life. Remember that now I wanted to teach you to beat the trap of avoidance. How.

By being proactive instead the trap of avoidance is you keep avoiding and evading and avoiding. Think of it like paying for your future on a credit card. You can have all the negativity that you owe for plus interest compounded and pretty soon it's going to be five 10 20 times 50 times worse than if you just dealt with it early. Deal with it now. Do it now. Proactive means to be active the moment you figure out that something is a problem now that could be even before it becomes a problem you could see where this is heading. You could read the writing on the wall and take care of it then. Or it's a small problem but you know it could get so much bigger. In therapy we used to say kill the monster while it's small so catch things early.

Take care of them when they're small. We used to say there was a time in the history of every problem when it was big enough to be seen but small enough to be dealt with easily. That's called being proactive. Avoidance is never ever going to work. It's childish it's do what this lady is. It's like covering your eyes and going La la la la la. I don't see anything. So therefore it must have gone away. A child will go and hide in a closet thinking that if they're in the closet they've left their problem behind. That's how childish avoidance is. Don't ever avoid your problems. They're never gonna get smaller. It won't be one time in a thousand that they go away but ninety nine times out of 100 they will get worse with simple avoidance and it will take so much more effort and so much more energy to take care of it. So be proactive. Deal with it early.

Crush it. Ask for help if you need help getting motivated, get out there and just do it. Journaling can be amazingly powerful and let me tell you why your thoughts and ideas look so different when you write them down on paper. So you'll write something down on a piece of paper. That's simply the thought going through your head and you'll look at it and look different to you. It won't look as bad on paper as it looked in your head or you'll write it down and you'll say Gosh as I look at that on paper I don't actually believe that or I don't think that's true or I noticed myself trying to write it down different on paper because it feels odd in a certain way like I'm overstating it I'm understating it it's not quite true it's a little embarrassing I don't want to put it that way because I don't want to be that kind of person.

There's a lot of influences that happen when the thoughts in your head get put down on paper that you'll be amazed by. You just gotta try it to learn about the power of journaling. Now here's the next power of a journal. Say your boss or somebody at work says something nasty to you but say it's your boss and the boss says hey you're a jerk or you did a terrible job on this. What you do is you'll run that a thousand times over in your head but you won't write it a thousand times on paper. You might write it down once or twice or three times. I've never seen a make over six that flipped the record where we're shooting for seven that's it. It stops that cycling that recycling of your pain over and over and over and over again in your head.

Simply by writing it down, that's an amazing power journey by itself. You will also think linearly as opposed to Circular Quay where you go over and over the same things by writing your thoughts, your ideas and your plans on paper. People don't loop on paper they loop in their head all the time they go back to old ideas. They go in circles they never go in circles and papers just one of those weird things is just activating a different part of your mind. So you're getting a different part of your genius going and you're leaving behind some of the delusion. A lot of things that you're delusional about in your life you won't write down on paper that way you become much more rational and less emotional on paper and therefore your thinking is clear on paper you can also review your thinking on paper you can notice the progress of your thinking on paper. There's a lot of power to journaling. Try it. Do it for a couple of weeks.

If you don't like it you can stop. But for a lot of people it's life changing. It's almost like being your own therapist in a book. You'll be able to see your own logic errors written in black and white in your own handwriting and you'll be able to correct them. Here's an old Buddhist Maxim. What do you have and what does that mean? It's literally the formula for happiness and satisfaction. What you have if you want the car that you have you're satisfied. If you don't want the car that you have then you feel like you have to go out and get a different car. Oh well now you got to spend a bunch of money on that car. You got this huge massive debt. You feel a little bit better in that car for 30 days 60 days 90 days.

It's the law of diminishing returns that pleasures dropping precipitously 90 days later. You are happier than when you had your old car. Now let me ask you: Did you have a 90 day loan? No. Therefore those payments are going to go out for two years four years six years. It's horrible and you don't feel any better and then you want another car and you're like oh my gosh you know before I had money in the bank I could've switched out my car anytime I want it you know. But now I got this loan and I don't have the money in the bank. I used it for the down payment. Now I'm poor. I put my financial health at risk and I don't feel any better in this car. And there's this other one that I want. Now you feel horrible.

So the Buddhists say it's insane to want something you don't have. It's simply a way for you to self torture yourself. It's you torturing yourself about what you don't have, the Buddhist saying, enjoy what you have. I have this car. This is a great car. A lot of people might not like my car but my car's paid for theirs is it. I actually bought my dad's old car. Now my dad has passed away recently but I have a lot of nice memories about that car and all the fun things we did in that car. You can't replace that car. Other people would look at and say you got money in your pocket. Why are you driving that piece of junk because it's not a bad car but it's not a luxury car. I could have.

So why am I driving around in it? I have no ego so I don't care about prestige symbols and luxury cars. I know I'm not going to be happier in one car than the other. It's where I go in the car, it's the memories I create in the car. It's how I feel in the car has nothing to do with the car. So I want the car I have now if I ever go out and buy another car I'll want that one. I'll have fond memories of the old one. I want the one that I'm in and I won't start wanting another car because that would be insane until I get to that next car. So this is part of reality therapy. Noticing what you have in appreciating what you have as opposed to comparing it to something you could have.

We call that the tyranny of better. There's always something better out there. You move from your apartment to a house and you say Oh and I got the house of my dreams. I'm so happy. Then you see a nicer house and you want that then you see a nicer house than that and you want that. Now you're into a multimillion dollar home. You say. Yeah but you know what. It's just not. If I had my own complex I would want to own Trump Tower. I want to own everybody's home. And then when you get done with that you're like well I want to own all of New York. Well, New York's kind of dirty and grungy. I want to own all of California. California's got too much smog. I want to own the whole United States.

You know I want to be ruler of the world. I want to own the entire planet. No no I want to own the universe. It goes for ever and ever and ever so wants are infinite true satisfaction comes from wanting what you have not the tyranny better not wanting more enjoying what you have I love this quote. I had this above my desk and if anybody ever said anything really stupid they started whining—or complaining. I would tap on that site. That was my only response style. I look over to them. I look over the side. I tap on it and I go back to work like they never said anything. And what did the sign say? It said any fool can whine—and complain and most Fools do so. Remember this quote. Write it down.

Tack it up on your wall, relax that when anybody out there in the universe you hear them whining—complaining you're simply hearing a fool and you know to listen to fools fools do what they do foolish things. You say well why are they whiny—equally. I don't know. That's what fools do. Looking at the sign again says it right there in black and white. Now having said this If you hear yourself whining—and complaining you're living great in your mind that this is what fools do you all want to be a fool you don't want to act fool if you don't want to take foolish actions you know to be seen as a fool and this will help you stop whining—and complaining because you don't want to be seen that way and you know it's wrong. Perfect sign I have perfect technique. Let it all go.

Now why do we say fools whine—and complain. Well a fool is not reality based. That's why they're so foolish they don't get the reality of the situation. They actually think. Hear this. They actually think that whining—or complaining are the same as taking actions. They sit around and they whine—and complain about the government and they think if they could just whine enough—enough or complain enough the government would mysteriously change. This is what we call therapeutic magical thinking. Why? Because it would literally take an act of magic if the wave your magic wand so that you're whining—you complaining would actually change anything.

It's the ultimate delusional thinking people will go out. They'll have problems with their boyfriend or problems with their girlfriend so they sit down with their friends and they whine—and complain about them actually thinking that whining—and complaining about your significant other to your friends will actually change your significant other. That's insane and people say well I'm not doing that I'm just doing that to vent and actually feel better if that venting actually worked. You'd feel better already. Why are you on a daily or weekly basis whining—complaining about your significant other over and over and over again for years.

Obviously this isn't a working man in fact most people are whining—complaining about something they're getting into that state. Notice how you feel when you win.—you complain. Do you feel better? Or do you feel worse? Do you feel more anxious or less you're going to see your anxiety level go up. You're going to feel your depression go up when you whine—or complain. Just another reason not to do it and shows that it's foolish to do it. Let it go. Don't lie don't—don't complain and don't spend time with people and whine—complain either. Why? Because they're fools.

Secondary Gains - Understanding - Choosing Your Emotions

Now I want to talk to you about the trap of secondary gains. This is a warning not a technique. See a lot of times our dysfunction actually has a function. What does that mean? It means it serves a purpose. It does something for us in a secondary fashion. So say you like this woman and you're shoving in one don't after the others. What's the primary game? Oh my God I don't, it tastes delicious. This is not rocket science. That's your primary game. That's your first game. What are your secondary gains? Well my sister Mary has a husband that likes to beat her and he's a sex addict and a—. So how does she keep him away from her? She eats a ton of doughnuts.

She's huge. She almost has to walk sideways to get through a door. Now her back hurts her knees. But believe me her husband doesn't want to go anywhere near her. She looks like holy hell. She used to be an attractive young woman. Then she met her husband Bob and now that's over. So primary game. Love the donuts. Eat the doughnuts. Secondary gain. Keep your crappy husband away from you. So a lot of things work like this in life. There's a lot of times where we're getting secondary gains. Here's another example of how secondary gains work. I had a client and she had fibro my LJM now fibromyalgia is a phantom pain syndrome.

We can't even tell if it's real or not. Matter of fact the way they diagnose it is the exact same way that we diagnose.

That's something somatic which means basically made up in your head locked in your head but not real. So that debate aside let's assume maybe it truly is neurological. Maybe it's a physiological disorder. Maybe she really does have this thing called fibromyalgia but she's still getting a lot of secondary gains and she would say I'm not getting any gains I just have a bunch of pain there is no pain no gain and pain right. So that's not absolutely true. She had a lot of secondary gains. First one is because she had fibromyalgia.

She was able to go on disability and never had to work again. That's a huge gain. I'd love to be able to just be semi retired and not have to work again. Wouldn't that be fantastic if I could just get a diagnosis that will allow me to stop working. Fantastic. I got a doctor's note. It's an excuse. It says I never have to work again but wonderful gain huge additional secondary gains any time she needs an excuse for something. Oh I can't do this, I can't do that, I can't stay. I've got to go. I don't want to do this. I don't want to do that. Why? Because my fibromyalgia is acting up she would get a lot of sympathy from her fibromyalgia.

Oh the pain and you'd understand and people would do special things for her and tell her how bad they felt for her and they'd give her a hug and all these wonderful things she would get a lot of attention for her fibro mile. It also excused why she had had all these problems in her life and all these things that went wrong for her. She could always blame it on her fibromyalgia. She wore this diagnosis like a blanket that she wrapped herself in. Poor me poor me. I have fibromyalgia and everybody needs to be good to me and everything's gotta go my way and nobody can say anything that I don't want them to say because I'll guilt them with my fibromyalgia.

She just wore this thing like a blanket. It was secondary gain secondary gain secondary gain. It went on and on and on and it was endless. That's why it was so difficult to treat her because I don't believe she had real fibromyalgia. She just had this pain that was very functional for her. So it was a somatic disorder really made up in her mind and she would never hear any of that and therefore didn't get any better because there were just so many secondary gains to keeping this somatic disorder rather than getting rid of it. It totally ruined treatment. There was just too much benefit too many people were buying into her game. So she ended up losing everybody around her.

So whenever you've got some kind of dysfunction look at what might be the secondary gains that I'm getting from this. If you can get rid of those secondary gains or at least see them for what they are which is pretty lame actually. You will be able to let them go and therefore you'll be more motivated to get out of the dysfunction that you have. It'll make it so much easier for you to leave this old dysfunction behind. Now one of the things that I want you to do in life is not to judge yourself by all the problems you have, all the challenges you have and all the horrible things that have happened in your life. What I want you to really judge yourself by is judge yourself by what you've survived.

Give yourself credit for that as much as you've achieved. It's more important what you've survived. So Judge yourself by two things. What I survived and what I've achieved, most people only give themselves credit for the things that they've achieved. Most of the things that they've survived were harder than the things that they achieved. You have to give yourself credit for both. And a lot of people haven't achieved much because they were so far behind the eight ball. They're dealing with anxiety, depression , low self-esteem, trauma phobias, you know, closed head injuries, mental retardation, all these different personality syndromes, all these tragedies that happen to them.

So they have a hard time achieving it's going to take them a while just to get back to zero so they can't judge themselves necessarily by what they achieved they didn't achieve as much as they wanted to in life because life didn't go the way they wanted it to. That's not their fault. That's not your fault. So to be fair to yourself it's okay to give you some credit for what you've achieved but also give yourself massive credit for what you've survived. It's only fair. Now I call this the power of understanding. It's very powerful. See, most problems are born out of ignorance. The challenge is we can't solve a problem that we don't know how to solve.

I used to ask this question and declined to say how many problems you can solve that you don't know how to solve. Correct answer. Zero. You can't solve a problem that you don't know how to solve so most problems are problems of ignorance. Do you know what the difference between ignorance and stupidity is? Ignorance is something I don't know. Once I do know I take action. Stupidity is. I didn't know. Now I do know and I don't take action now you're just stupid OK. It's OK to be ignorant, it's not OK to be stupid. What's the difference? You take action. So go out there, find a solution and take massive action. You have to look at the problem. Ask for help. Read the self-help books, check on youtube and google it.

Get therapy. Whatever you have to do so that you're no longer ignorant about the problem. You know the solution. And then go out and take massive action. And don't blame yourself. Remember the whole period, the whole time in which you could not solve the problem. It was impossible. You didn't know how. Let go of all that guilt. So the guilt is not your fault. Let it go but it is your responsibility to go out and find a solution. Today. Now here's another secret of psychology that most people don't know is that almost every single human action is based on how we see ourselves and the world. This is almost like the logic premise that we function from. If you think you can or you think you can't you're right. I love that old quote.

That's a quote about how you see yourself if you think you can. You can if you think you can't you can't. You're setting a glass floor and a glass ceiling for yourself. You're determining by the way you look at yourself what things you can do and can't do. You do this in every single area of your life and most of it is just a story. It's just an image that you have of yourself that maybe you've been true at one time but isn't necessarily true today. You can see how people can act wildly differently under hypnosis. What does hypnosis do? It removes that story and simply has you perform the way you're asked to perform versus the way you see yourself performing in your story.

It removes the story and instantly people can do things that they thought they couldn't do simple. Now we also take actions based on how we see the world. So not necessarily just ourselves but the world. If we think the world is a safe place then we're going to go out and we're gonna do things and we're gonna be adventurous. Why? Because it's safe to do those things. If we think we're safe we'll take certain risks. Why? Because it doesn't seem as risky to us. We know that even if things go bad will somehow pull it out. If you see the world is scary you're not going to venture out there and you're not going to take risks because you think if you take the risk and you lose you can never make up for that loss or the loss is gonna be a crushing or devastating war.

You just can't recover from it or be so embarrassed. You can't possibly do that. That's a view of the world. So I want you to know that a lot of what you think you can do or not do is based on your view of the world or the view of yourself in that most of that view is just an opinion. It's illusionary, break free of the illusion and you will gain new talents, new abilities, new perspectives and feel totally different about yourself and the world. The way you think about yourself is the way you feel about yourself, the way you think about the world is the way you feel about the world. Meditate on it for a while. Change either those perspectives or more powerfully change them both in. Everything will change for you. Now here's what I want you to do. I want you to learn to act but don't react.

Don't live in reaction. Think of it this way. Find the unnecessary step. You have a problem. Then you feel bad about it and then you solve the problem. What's the unnecessary step of feeling bad about it? You have to have the problem. The problem really occurred. It exists. That has to be there. Feeling bad doesn't have to exist but because you have the problem that's real you also have to solve it. So the problem is Israel. Solution Israel. They're both necessary. Feeling bad in between worrying kvetching draining yourself whining—complaining. These are all unnecessary steps.

You are gonna feel so much better in life if you simply go from problem to solution problem to solution. ACTs don't react or keep the reaction minimal. Shrink it down to its proper size. Its proper size is zero but on a scale of 1 to 10 it should never be a 10. Could be like one , two or three. And even then it should fade quickly back into the solution they say when I stop focusing on the problem and I start focusing on a solution. The problem goes away so whenever you have a problem instead of going into reactions that are feeling bad. Try to get past that and immediately go into the solution and as you're solving it it's hard to go back and feel bad because as you're solving it you're seeing it go away so you can't put in a lot of attention or a lot of energy into something that's going away.

But if you're if you have a problem and then you get wrapped up in the emotion and the emotion is so intense that you don't take any action and it almost makes you want to move away from the solution because the solution would be painful. You will sit in that painful emotion for a long period of time. Some people will do it until they get so depressed that the solution seems impossible and they've drained off all their energy and now they have no energy to get into the solution and solve the problem. Makes sense. Now this is going to sound strange to a lot of people. I want you to learn how to choose your emotions. Let me ask a question. Did you know that your emotions are actually a choice a lot of people think oh my emotions just happen to me.

Not necessarily. You could have the same thing happen to three different people and they would act three different ways. Why? Well one based on their old programming or two they chose a different way of looking at it and therefore they created a different emotion. We talked about this when we talked about reframing how you look at something. Now you can also simply choose the emotion when you have a chapter to do. You can choose to be scared or choose to be excited. Two different choices, two different experiences. Your emotions are a choice. Think of it this way. Somebody is late for something. You can choose to worry about that person. Oh my God what happened to them or be angry. They don't value my time.

They're late. I'm always on time. Why do they have to be late? Seeing your emotions is a choice now a lot of times that choice is based on how you picture what's going on. You picture somebody disrespecting you or you picture somebody in trouble and then the natural emotion follows.

So one way to choose emotions is simply to choose to feel one way versus the other and the other way to change the emotion is to choose how to look at a situation because there's an infinite number of ways to look at the same situation. So these are the two ways that you can actually learn how to choose your emotions. So take some time to think about what I've said, try it out in a couple of different scenarios, meditate on it, try it, practice and brainstorm how you can do it.

Don't let this one chapter by saying Oh I got it. This is one we have to play with for a while to realize that you can actually choose your emotions. And until you do it in life and you pick between two different emotions and you do this several times in your life to give yourself good powerful references that you actually are choosing. You have examples of times where you've chosen it. It won't be real for you. You can't understand this intellectually. You have to understand this experientially by doing it now. I'm gonna teach you the law of reciprocity and reflection. You're kind of the same thing. The law of reciprocity says that if I do something nice for you you're going to want to do the same thing back.

So if I do something nice for you you want to do the same thing back or a little bit more reciprocity also works in the negative if I do something nasty to you. You want to also do something nasty back plus a little bit more but it's always giving back in like plus a little bit more. That's how the law of reciprocity works. The law of reflection says that what you give out into the universe comes back to you if you look at somebody with a smile. You notice they tend to smile back.

You give somebody a dirty look. They tend to give you a dirty look back or they look confused. Why is this person doing this? But it's one of the others. So we look at life as a mirror and say why are people so negative. Well a lot of times people that say why are people so negative when you read them in their interactions.

That's what they're putting out to the universe and it's getting reflected back. They're acting negative and then they wonder why all this negativity is coming back. So reciprocity and reflection are kind of two ways to say almost the same thing. There's a fundamental force out there. It's just a law of nature that what you put out there comes back to you. So the way that we use this to feel better is to give the feelings to others that you want. If I want people to be nicer to me I'm going to be nicer to them. If I want people to be more loving towards me I want to be more loving towards them even if I want to create more fun. If I tell more jokes and I have more fun with people they're going to start doing that back.

People love to follow this law. Reciprocity is always there. If I'm more generous with my friends you know nine nine times out of 100 they're going to be more generous with me. So if you want to create the kind of life, the kind of environment, the kind of friendships, the kind of relationships that you want. Do what I call. Going first. Show them what you want. You want them to treat you in more respect. You give them more respect. You want them to be more loving, you be more loving towards them. This will work about 99 percent of the time. So put out there into the world what you want the world to give back to you and you'll do fantastic.

Emotional Timer" - Trust - Fairness - ZEN

Let me ask you a question. How long should an emotion last? It's a great question. A lot of people have different timers on how long their emotions should last. I literally call it an emotional timer. Some people think if somebody says something nasty to you you should let it last five minutes. Other people say five hours five days five years. Some people say forever given the fact that we're making up this number, why don't we make it a number that we're happier with. Try to drop your number down as low as you can get it. Remember holding a resentment is like taking poison thinking the other person will die.

It only hurts you. So remember this concept, it's just an idea in your head how long it should last. So ask yourself what would be the appropriate amount of time to hurt myself because of somebody else's action correct number zero. And try to get as close to that number as you can. Here's another great concept. Learn to think and feel rationally rationality reality. What a concept. Use your intellect not emotion over intellect but intellect over emotion intellect controlling emotion look at things rationally instead of emotionally and you drain the emotional content out of it. Be objective. Always try to look at things that are happening in your life as if you could step out and look at them from the outside.

So you're looking at these as if they're happening to somebody else that's looking at it intellectually focusing on the solution instead of the emotional content is thinking rationally. All these things drop down the emotionality, the negative emotions that you're feeling as you're going through the process and as you lower the emotions and raise the intellect. Solutions come in because you're kicking in your logical brain which is the part that solves problems instead of your emotional centers which sit in problems breaking news. Life's not a fair suggestion. Get over it. Just get over it. Life is never gonna be fair. Here's what I tell my clients about fair.

When you're a young kid between 0 and somewhere between the age of 16 and 20 people run around society. Teachers RUN AROUND. EVERYBODY RUNS AROUND YOUR PARENTS run around your friends run around everybody running around trying to make life fair for you but then it's never fair again. This probably isn't a good way to set kids up but there it is. So a lot of people go through life with delusion thinking that life should be fair and people say oh Mr. I don't I don't believe that life should be fair. Then why do you get upset when it isn't the only way you can actually get upset when life isn't fair that you can be mad about if you thought it should be fair. It wasn't.

And now you're mad. Otherwise life wasn't fair. I thought life wasn't gonna be fair and it wasn't. Huh. Perfect. There's nothing to get upset about. It's only when you think life should be fair and then it's not that you get mad. So if something happens in your life and you get upset about it don't tell me that you know life isn't fair. You don't. You may know on an intellectual level but on an emotional level you're thinking about it like that young child where everybody's running around and trying to make it better. So I tell my clients to go to the fair in Tampa. It's awesome at this fair they got cotton candy and they've got Ferris wheels and they've got hot dogs and drumsticks and log rolling and big pigs you can play with all kinds of fun events and games and all kinds of shows. It's amazing you should go to that fair.

Why? Because that's the only fair you're gonna see all year. The rest of the year there is no fair. Life is not fair. Take fairness out of your mind, it's an absurd idea. Get rid of it once you get rid of it. You're gonna feel a thousand percent better here's an interesting thing. Trust versus mistrust people think. Trust is all about the other person. My goodness can I trust them or can I trust them. No. Trust isn't about them, it's about you. It's about you, not the other person. The question isn't whether or not you can trust the other person. The question is can I trust my ability to assess. Is the other person trustworthy? They're either trustworthy or they're not.

The only time it impacts me is when I can't assess properly if I know something's going to lie to me or cheat on me or do me dirty and I know that. Then I can take the appropriate steps and they really don't do anything negative in my life. That's perfect. I can avoid this person. I just don't trust them in that area. Now there's some people you can trust in certain areas. There's some people I'll trust with my car but I wouldn't trust him with my girlfriend because other people that I would trust with my girlfriend. But I probably wouldn't lend him my car. See what I'm saying. So trust is about your ability to assess the other person. Or it may even be trust issues that you have. Either way trust is about you not about the other person.

People are going to be the way they are. Your job is to get better at detecting liars , detecting people that aren't trustworthy. Being accurate in your assessments trusting people that you can trust because if you don't trust people you can trust that'll hurt your life in not trusting the people that you can't really trust that will always boil down to assessment. There's a great book called Never be lied to again. You should read that one and other ones by that author. He has a lot of different literature and a lot of great self-help books on how to detect how people are thinking and why they're doing things. So it's a great book to read and it will help you get those better assessment skills.

Now if you want to be able to handle your emotions you've gotta get behind the wheel. What I mean by getting behind the wheel well we can't always pick the thoughts that come into our head and therefore the emotions that are attached to them but you can't steer them. That's what I mean by getting behind the wheel. Your thoughts are going to move you in certain directions towards the positive towards the negatives towards fear towards anxiety towards depression. You're going to see them going in that direction. And what I want you to do is when you see him going in the wrong direction. I want you to start to turn it around. Catch it early. Catch it often when you're feeling negatively.

You simply went in the wrong direction and depending upon the severity how bad it feels. You went too far in that direction. How do you solve it? Turn around. Go in the opposite direction and start moving in the positive direction that you want to go to see your brain will move you in a certain direction and unless you intercede, unless you jump in and say I'm actually gonna take control of my own thought process as my own emotions. It'll just take you wherever it wants to. And by default it tends to move towards the negative. It's just how the human brain is hardwired. It's almost as if you had a car with a bad alignment and always went to the left OK. If you don't want to go to the left all the time and you gotta constantly hold on to the wheel or be readjusting.

That's what I mean by steering your emotions. You can do it but you've got to be aware of this process. Be mindful of what's going on for your emotions and take corrective actions to move your thoughts in the direction you want them to go. Now here's a little bit of Zen philosophy and I put the words up. Good bad maybe. What does that mean? It means the hardest thing in the mind is to leave a question mark. The mind hates a vacuum. In nature a vacuum will suck in anything. So it's hard to leave that vacuum, that empty space in your mind. I'm not going to decide just yet. Your brain likes to decide instantly like a placeholder like a vacuum it will suck something in. Unfortunately it's not always true.

So true genius is the ability to say I'm thinking about a certain thing a certain way but it's just a placeholder. I could be right. I could be wrong. I may need to adjust that to keep a question mark next to everything in your mind that you believe. Now there's the old Zen story about good, bad and maybe a gentleman. He has a loving family, his wife and his son and he has a couple of horses in one day. The horses are able to kick at the barn door and they kick it open and they run off and the guy loses his two horses. Well that was pretty much everything it had. And the neighbors come and they say oh my god what horrible luck. That's really bad luck.

I'm so sorry for you and the farmer simply says good luck bad luck. I don't know, maybe neighbors look kind of strange and they walk off a couple of days later. Those horses met up with some wild stags and they all came back home in three wild stags came back with the original two horses. Now the guy went from two horses to five horses. Neighbors come by and say This is fantastic. You've had such great luck. This is good luck. Farmer says good luck bad luck. Maybe I don't know if neighbors will look at him again like he's crazy a couple of days later. He's trying to tame one of the horses and he gets thrown and he breaks his leg. Neighbors come by.

Oh my God what bad luck. This is horrible. Palmer says good luck bad luck. Maybe I don't know if neighbors look at him again like he's crazy. A couple of days later the military comes by and they're grabbing every male child of military age whose son has that able body. They see his broken leg and they pass him by. Everybody that got taken in the military service about 90 percent of them died neighbors came by said Oh you're so fortunate. They took our sons. They left yours. You're so lucky and the farmer says good luck bad luck maybe I don't know. Now that's the end of the story but the story could go on and on and on. We don't know until everything is all done which means we're done.

If something was good or bad it could be either so if you believe something's good or bad. Remember to keep a question mark there because the real answer is maybe here's an interesting philosophy. Bad times are actually good. Why? Because they make us stronger. Think of it this way less Brown always says in the good times. You put it in your pocket in the hard times you put in your heart which means when things go great you profit from them. When things go bad you strengthen from that. That's why you can always take the bad things that happen and use them to make yourself stronger.

You can also take the bad times and figure out how not to have them again in the future. Learn from your mistakes and then they make you stronger next time where you don't have to be stronger because you can completely avoid it. Also you can help out other people that are about to go through these bad times or are going through these bad times and now because you were there before them. You know the way out. I was very impressed with this when I first started counseling alcoholics and addicts about all these horrible horrible things they had gone through. They saw them as gifts. Why? Because they had gone through these things. They could show other recovering addicts how to avoid them or how to overcome them.

Their pain had actually become something that they could use to help other people. So something that had been horrible in their lives was actually giving them power and helping other people. That's so beautiful. If you look at your challenges, past , present and future in a way that they're going to strengthen you, they're going to teach you how to avoid them in the future. They're going to make you stronger and more capable you're going to learn something in this area and that you're going to be able to share that knowledge to help somebody else. This can make a lot of the bad times into good times for you. Let me ask you a question.

Are you a pessimist? If so, here's what I want you to do: slap yourself. Who sold you on that plan and why did you listen to him? A lot of people are pessimists thinking they're realists. Being a pessimist is about the dumbest thing you can do. The optimists feel fantastic while a pessimist feels horrible their entire life. You can't win by feeling horrible your entire life. This is a plan of an idiot now an optimist is not naive. They know there's challenges out there and they know how to avoid those challenges. They just maintain a positive attitude. In the meantime the pessimist thinks the optimist doesn't know that these problems are out there. That's how stupid the pessimist is. So I don't know who sold you on this plan but you should hunt him down and give him a good beating. Don't listen to them any more.

Get out of pessimism. Get into optimism. Feel better every single day. Your job in life is not to feel bad. Your job is to maximize your joy in life and to bring other people with you. The exact opposite of what a pessimist does. A pessimist feels bad and then invites other people to join them. Pure utter insanity. If you're pessimistic in any way shape or form let it go. I like to think I was optimistic but as I listened to my language and the directions I went into. We talked about steering your emotions and steering your thoughts. I notice that even though I was pretty much an optimist. A lot of times I would steer into pessimism and I would have to catch myself and realize this is stupid.

Even if you're only doing it part time you know you're supposed to feel good all the time. At least try to move in that direction so catch yourself stop yourself move back in the positive direction. Now one of the ways you can do that is through your power of choice. You literally get to choose what you're going to do. You can choose to hurt people or heal people to hate people or love people to talk or to listen to shrink or to grow to deny or to accept to hold on to or to release to go for the negative or go for the positive to be telling or to be teaching to attack or to help to be egotistical or to learn. So a lot of your life is going to be as you look at these two lists which side you choose from and these are just examples. We can all make very long lists like this. Make sure you're picking from the right pile.

GIGO - Meditation - Escape - Things that Don't Exist

Now this seems like a simple tip but it's going to affect you profoundly short term and long term. Let's talk about the short term ego as an old acronym. It was originally used by I.T. people garbage in garbage out. If you program in garbage garbage comes back out. Computers can only put out what you put in your brain just like a computer. Whatever you put in. That's what I'll come out with. You put great things in great things that come out. You put crap in crapola come out. Be very careful what you put in your brain. Don't fill it with rubbish like negative news and thoughts about angry or negative people.

You know, look out in the environment and put great things into your mind. Positive things that you write optimistic things in your mind, things that are moving toward your goal that make you happy in the short term will change your state because what you focus on you get more of. So this information is coming in. If you're putting in great positive information, great positive inputs, the output which is your emotions are also going to feel absolutely fantastic. Now that's in the short term instantly literally as you're doing it. It's creating this positive state change. The second thing is as you fill your brain with this you'll have lots and lots of positive references.

You'll have been keeping your mind positive for a long period of time. This will sink into your subconscious and it will keep you positive even in the down times if you keep filling it with enough positive stuff. Eventually what will happen is positivity and feeling good will literally get hard wired into your neurons into your brain and will become a habit. It'll be your default just like depressed people that are constantly bringing in depressing thoughts. They feel depressed at the moment. Long term they feel depressed. It sinks into the subconscious and becomes their default. Whenever they say I don't know how to feel, they feel bad. So there's nothing wrong with this system. You just have to use it in the positive. If you've got depression you already know how it works.

If you've got anxiety you already know how it works. It's based on the inputs. So this seems like a simple strategy, a simple technique and that's what's great about it. It is simple but it's also amazingly powerful in some ways. If this is all that you did this in and of itself would be a great therapy and a great way to change your mental state both short term and long term it's absolutely fantastic. And it's absolutely crucial if you try all the other strategies that you keep filling your mind full of negative rubbish you're going to have a hard time feeling better in life. Why? Because you're constantly working against yourself. So be very careful about your inputs, what you read on TV, what you read in magazines , friends , things that you read, any kind of mental input things that you listen to, maybe on the radio. Be very careful what you're inputting into your brain.

Remember that's what's going to come back out. You may be listening to a radio show and say oh they're just whining and complaining about this person to the other person. No it's pure bile it's negativity and it's going into your brain. Think of this as the analogy of you are what you eat which means whatever you consume into your body is transformed into your body and that's how your body comes out. Same thing with your brain. What you put into your brain transforms your brain and that's how your brain ends up. So no it's not negativity about somebody else. It ends up landing on you. All inputs affect you, you or somebody else could be sitting there talking negatively about somebody else and all your brain hears is negativity negativity negativity and says OK I'll start programming that negativity and be very careful.

So take this tip very seriously, review it and make sure to check yourself throughout the day that you are putting the right inputs in meditation is something I absolutely love. Now a lot of people don't even know what meditation is. I highly recommend that you do it live with somebody to learn how to get into the proper state. So there's lots of places out there that would give low cost no cost meditation Books or at least read some youtube chapters on it so you can have a real live human being kind of walk you through the experience. But at the fundamental core meditation is as simple as reducing your thinking down to one steady thought, not this constant stream of multi-tasking chatter that your brain normally does but getting down to reduce stimulus getting into a sleep-like state almost like you're ready to drift off to sleep at night. That's what meditation is.

It reduces the chatter and it gets your brain into the right alpha beta state to be able to accept programming by you and from you and incorporate it. This is a way to get around the conscious brain and get closer to the unconscious brain. That's literally what I mean when I say it's like when you drift off to sleep when you drift off to sleep What are you doing. You're going from the conscious to the unconscious. Now if you fall asleep you're unconscious, if you're fully awake and you're not in that dreamlike state then you're fully conscious and you're talking to the conscious mind. We want to get into that in-between state where we're both conscious and unconscious.

Here's what we're saying: getting into the unconscious mind we'll put whatever you program into it on autopilot and we'll get into those deeper recesses that are sometimes hard to get to. Sometimes people say I feel bad. I don't know why. It's probable that you're not reading your inputs like we just talked about garbage in garbage out. That's one cause of that. The other causes old paint, old negativity bubbling up through the unconscious and making you feel bad and you don't know where it came from because you're like Hey I wasn't putting in bad inputs and yet I feel bad PTSD is all about stuff bubbling up from the unconscious. So meditation is literally a way to get into that dreamlike state.

Relax yourself completely it feels fantastic and then go ahead and give yourself suggestions. Now when you're giving suggestions you have to give yourself positive suggestions. Things like I'm relaxed. I'm positive. I'm at peace. My memory is increasing and my weight is dropping. I feel healthy and good about my life. Every day new good things are coming into my life and I keep a positive mindset. Those are all good positive things that you can program into the brain just as examples. Think of it like self hypnosis where you can literally hypnotize yourself, get into that dream-like state and then put in suggestions. Now there's a hypnosis tape for virtually everything but what they'll tell you and I believe it's true is that hypnosis tapes never program a negative so don't say stop worrying stop worrying stop worrying.

The stop is a negative in your brain. Here's worrying worrying worrying when you say don't think about this it here. Think about this. So say you wanted to get away from a thought or get away from something like you want to get away from the anxiety. You don't say stop feeling anxious. You say I'm releasing all anxiety now anxiety is fleeing my body or even better is to put myself in the actual state that you want. I feel relaxed and free at peace. That's the opposite of anxiety. And it's a positive program. So meditation is a great way to slow down that busy thought. Traffic within your head. It's a great way to practice mental control. This will help you tremendously with some of the techniques that we've gone over like focusing your thoughts.

Being able to manage what you focus on is why meditation is literally the practice of controlling your mind when you first start trying to meditate. You'll notice that your brain fights you. Why? Because it's not under your control yet you've never practiced controlling your mind. So it'll fight you over and over and over again but as you fight with your brain to try to get it to work with you you will learn specific tool strategies and techniques for how to get your brain to work with you and get it under your control so that now you're a team instead of almost an opposition which isn't a good position to be in. So meditation is a very powerful technique. It's great for programming and it's great for relieving stress and gaining the abilities you want to have so you can use it to lose weight, improve your memory, and improve your relationships. I always use it for healing.

I use it for relaxation. There's a dozen or more different things that you can use it for dozens is probably understating it there's literally hundreds of things that you can use it for. You simply have to say what is within the ability of my mind to grant me and then ask for that thing in a positive fashion. Do it repeatedly because remembering the subconscious is a little bit slow. You might have to do it 10, 20 , 30 times , that's OK. Do it once a day for 10 minutes. Program it in there somewhere between maybe a week and four weeks. Boom it'll be yours. Lock it in forever. That's beautiful. Now I use this phrase: don't be your own jailer. A lot of people blame themselves for certain things or they keep repeating the past. They refuse to release the past; they keep running it like an old movie in their head that literally traps them in their own pain.

You have to forgive yourself and let go with the past. I remember one client saying to me I said what was one of the best things you ever learn in treatment. He said, " , I don't know if you said it to one of the other clients, but somebody said yesterday's not getting any better and what that said to me is that the past is the perfect preservative. It never gets any better. So you don't go back and try to fix the past or heal the past. It's never going away. You release yourself from the past, you walk away from your past, you restart your life, you move forward, you let it go. You do that by simply letting go. And by forgiving yourself you release the past. That's how you'll lighten the load. Not trying to fix the past is never going to get any better.

Not by reviewing the past it's never going to look any different. It might look a little worse over time letting go and forgiving yourself so don't be the person that causes their own pain that traps themselves in the pain. Don't be your own jailer, forgive yourself, let it go. You would do this for a good friend. You would never say to a friend Oh you're bad forever because you did such and such. Now you'd say hey give yourself a break. You need to be a good friend to yourself, maybe externalize yourself, see yourself as a good friend outside yourself and then forgive yourself. Sometimes that works for people but think would I hold this against my best friend if you wouldn't then let it go. And if you would let it go anyways because it just means you're a bad friend.

We should all let go of the past because remember the past doesn't exist. We can start our life over from here forward. It doesn't matter if we ever did anything bad in the past. If you're not going to do it again in the future then you're free to let it go. And this is one of the major ways that you release yourself from old pain. So this is not a small thing you have to forgive yourself to release the past. And sometimes you have to forgive others to release the past because you're holding on to these things because you want them to apologize. It's not about them apologizing. It's about you getting rid of the pain. They don't have to apologize for that. You can let it go.

If somebody insults me they can apologize or not apologize. I always let go of the pain. I always let it go. Why? Because it only hurts me and I let it go because I can't. Why would I ever sit there in pain? Day after day after day waiting for an apology when at the end of the day I'm the one that lets it go anyways and I can instantly let it go. Friendship friends are very powerful healers. Just being around good people is healing. You know a lot of people believe it's a metaphysical thing you're transferring energy and all that positive energy is floating around and going through you. Who knows from a physics perspective is a little bit of evidence for that. Otherwise it just sounds a little fluffy to me. But hey go for it.

But psychologically being around positive people getting all those positive inputs that we've been talking about tonight is even just healing touch. Giving them a hug slapping him on the back and a handshake. Anything being able to share your lives with people. I know my life isn't great until I share something that was great that happened. I share it with my wife. It's kind of nice when it happens but it's wonderful like I share with my wife. So sharing it with your significant other being around good friends these are really good forms of medicine. It will literally heal your mind, your spirit, whatever. It's absolutely fantastic. So keep good people around you, get rid of all the negative people and spend time with good friends. It's amazingly uplifting.

It works instantly. That friendship is a positive reference, a positive memory in your mind. It sinks into your unconscious and is there like a store of energy like a reserve. It's one of those positive things you can put into your unconscious mind that will support you during the down times. Now here's something fascinating. Let me give you a nice list of things that actually don't exist and this is a great way to think about it. If I said once you run outside and go to a store go wherever you want and get me a twelve pound bag of anxiety where would you go. You can't get a bag of anxiety because anxiety doesn't exist and nobody is handing it out. Same thing for depression.

Depression doesn't actually exist. This is one of the reasons why people have such a hard time with anxiety and depression. You are literally fighting something that doesn't exist. It's a story. It's a work of fiction. That kind of story in your mind. That's all it is. Your anxiety and your depression, your fears, your guilt, your traumas, all your thoughts about the past. They literally don't exist except as a memory or as a thought in your head. So I like people to think about this way and to rehearse this idea to let it sink into the unconscious because this will help the unconscious release it that it doesn't really exist. We get so wrapped up in our past and our trauma and our anxiety and our depression and all our thoughts we think thoughts or things they're not like electrons.

They're like the Internet. It's flowing through the cable all the time but it really doesn't exist. It's something that exists when you activate it so you can activate your anxiety and it will seem very real. You can activate your depression and it will seem very real. You can activate your trauma. It'll seem very real. You can activate your fear and it will seem very real because it has a huge impact on you but it's fiction again. Your anxiety or depression, your past, your fear, your guilt, your trauma. We keep going down through the list all these things physically don't exist. This is one of the reasons you have to learn how to control them and not activate them. And when they come, learn how to let them go.

They basically feed off your thoughts, your thoughts, your feet activate them, your thoughts feed them, your thoughts help them to grow and you can do the opposite. You can starve them. You can not activate them. You can change the thoughts and you will wipe these things out but just remember they physically don't exist. They're just a story you have in your head and you seriously need to change that story. And these things never have control over you, you have control over them. But much like you have control over your own mind but you haven't practiced the control of your mind like we were talking about in the meditation because you haven't practiced control over these things. They run away with you. You haven't learned how to control them. But remember they don't exist.

What Next

Now if you want to recover guess what. You gotta have a recovery plan. And what's a recovery plan? A recovery plan is a plan for massive action. Remember nobody is coming to the rescue, this chapter is the rescue. It should lead you to everything else that you need. One of the things that I've always been very proud of is when I finish counseling a person they continue to get better even after they leave me. Why? Because I've taught them how to teach themselves. And I've also given them so many tips, strategies , tools , techniques that they couldn't possibly ever complete them within our counseling period. I might be with them for a month or two but I probably gave them somewhere between a year to five years worth of stuff to do to improve their life.

So keep going over this chapter and looking at different ways that you can change your life. So take one tool. One strategy, one technique. Live with it for a few days, maybe even a couple of weeks if it's a really powerful one. Ingrain that. Make sure you've got it nailed down so that you use that tool and strategy. That technique is almost reflexive. Now let's go back to recovery plans. If you've got depression you need to have a depression recovery plan. What's it going to look like? Well it's going to look like going through this chapter and taking every depression tool strategy and technique and start applying those. But you may also start a recovery plan for depression. Beyond that you may want to say OK what self-help books are out there for depression specifically what youtube chapters.

Could I read those who are depressed, specifically learning new strategies and tools every day? What other chapter Books could I take that are specific to depression. What changes in my life can I make? Because it's hard to get past depression when you're sitting in an environment with a lifestyle the way that your life is set up to literally cause depression. That becomes part of the action plan. How can I bring in good positive people in my life to help me get past the depression and to keep a positive flow of energy going in my life. So go down each and every area and look at how I can create more recovery, more recovery, more recovery. What do I need to learn?

What do I need to do and what actions do I need to take? If you work on that plant you develop that plan. You take massive action on that plan then you're going to do absolutely fantastic. Your anxiety or depression, your low self-esteem whatever your issue is can not survive your focused attention on defeating it. Remember it's your anxiety, your depression, your low self-esteem. These are things that don't exist. You're creating them. You can create them in the same system used to say to get massively depressed is the same one that people used to be massively happy. It's just different inputs. So a lot of the tools that you think you need you already use them to make yourself feel rotten.

You can use the exact same strategies. There's nothing wrong with the strategies they clearly work to make yourself feel fantastic. So get a plan. Write it down, scratch it out on paper, and start doing a little bit every day. No pressure if you can survive things getting worse and worse like they have over time. You can survive things getting better and better. It's a beautiful progression to read so work on your action plan every day. Even if it's just for five minutes every day, take a positive action that'll ingrain into your mind consciously in the moment and subconsciously long term that I am going to beat this thing. This thing is not going to beat me. I am going to have that freedom from pain that I want. I'm going to have joy and vitality and a life second to none.

That's my wish for you. But it takes action. I love this acronym. It's called the how acronym stands for honesty, openness and willingness. You're out there in a place called the School of Life. And it's always giving you different lessons. And if you're honest with yourself you don't kid yourself. You don't lie to yourself. You don't shift it. You don't use your biases and your prejudices and your histories. You just honestly let the lessons in you're open to hearing them and you're willing to make changes based on what you're seeing. You're being a good student of life then life is going to give you a series of lessons and you can learn from them.

Make sure you take away the right lessons. When somebody says something nasty to you that doesn't mean you're a bad person and other people are bad people and life is horrible. It means that when people are in pain they leak it out on you and you can see that person is hurt or injured. That's the correct lesson. Make sure you're getting the right lesson. The lesson is I'm strong, I can take it. The lesson is this is an opportunity for me to practice letting these things go. Thank you for that opportunity. I can't practice it unless you give me something to practice on. This person is not your enemy, they're your teacher. Honesty, openness, and willingness are great techniques to learn from life, which is how we do most of our learning anyways experientially out there in the field dealing with life.

Make sure that you're grabbing the right lessons and looking at things the right way. Saying that what I'm learning is helping me or hurting me is moving me in the right direction or the wrong direction. It's moving you in the right direction. You probably got the right lesson. If it's moving you in the wrong direction. Look at it again because 99 percent of the time you got the law the wrong lesson. Switch it out now let me ask you this: what do you need to let go of that you're still holding on to whatever it is. It's not really a part of you letting it go, it's hurting you. Let me ask you something. How do you let something go let's say you have a rock in your hand or a hot coal. You want to let go of it. How do you let go of it? You simply release it.

You let go. When you become willing to unclench your fist to open your hand it's your willingness to let go that allows these things to go away. A lot of people are waiting. Hoping it'll go away. They're hoping time will make it go away. If time made it go away there probably would be nobody reading this Book there'll be nobody reading this Book. How many things have you been holding onto that you've been holding on to for five 10 15 20 30 40 for some people 50 60 70 years. Waiting is not how you let go. It's your willingness to let it go. You've got to get a peace deal. And letting go practice letting go meditate on letting go. Notice as you're holding on to it. What am I doing at this moment as I'm holding onto it?

How am I sustaining this pain, not the experience of the pain not focusing on the feeling of the pain but how I'm holding onto it, how I'm creating it, how I'm supplying it with energy. These are the things that keep it in your press. These are the things that keep it in your mind and do the opposite. And that's how you let go. Letting go is amazingly free. Now we've talked about this a bit before the power of positive thinking. You've a particular activator in your brain. It's a little shrimp sized mechanism and it's shoved up in between the folds in the center of your brain down at the bottom and whatever you focus on triggers the rectangular activator.

The particular activator is a scanner. It will go through whatever you're focusing on. It will go through the environment, scan the environment and find things that relate to that. So when you'll be a negative it tries to scan the environment and says oh I guess we're looking for negative things. And it scans the environment and looks for negative things. When you think about positive things it scans the environment and tries to find positive things. So the particular activator kind of does two things. It focuses on and finds more things in the environment based on whatever you're focusing on. And it supports your ideas and your goals. If your goal is to be depressed it'll say yes sir yes ma'am I will get right on it and I will find all kinds of things that will support you in your goal to be depressed.

But if your goal is to be happy, to be serene, to have a great day, it will scan the environment and find things that support that and give you ideas and thoughts and memories that support that for most of us. We've been using our particular activities the wrong way. Why? Because we didn't even know that it existed. Now you know it's a tool now you know it's a resource now that you know how this system works. You can begin using it in your favor. Now as much as the particular activator grabs things from the environment that support whatever you're thinking on positive or negative it's also a deletion key. It deletes anything that doesn't match what you're thinking about what you're focusing on.

So if you're focusing on the positive, not only will it scan the environment and grab all the positive things, it will actively block out the negative things. This is why depression is so powerful when you focus on negative things. It not only scans for the pause for the negative things that are out there to support your depression. It blocks out all the positive things that could come in and ruin a perfectly good depression. So nothing wrong with a device except how you're using it. You know a car can drive you where you want to go or you can drive it into a tree. In either case the vehicle is functioning perfectly.

One I'll help you. One will hurt you. It's not a tool. It's how you're using it. Make sure you're using your particular activator, your ability to focus on things and using it the proper way. Now here's a key technique you really seriously need to change people, places and things that are negative in your life. Negative people can literally suck the life out of you. So get rid of all the negative people and never look back and say I wish I waited longer to get rid of this negative person get rid of them with prejudice literally as if in this picture they were a vampire in your life they were going to kill you because they literally are they're destroying the joy in your life and that's your only reason for living is to enjoy life.

It's your purpose. So get back to your purpose. Now we're looking at people, places and things. So there's positive people there's negative people had more positive people were the negative people there's positive places places that make you feel good that are serene that are helpful is also negative places places like bars that could be really negative where negative people hang out is also negative things there's positive books and there's negative books those are things there's things in your life that help you and hurt you that are things you know a it is a nice treat once in a while but that can also be a negative thing if you keep it in the house and you're on a diet you know a vegetable in that case would be a positive thing.

You know a low calorie substitute snack would be a positive thing. Keeping things around your house that reminds you of good times are positive things. Negative things are things that bring back old negative memories. So remember people, places and things that your action list goes through in your life. Start removing the negative and start adding the positive and you'll be amazed before you're halfway done at what a huge state change happens. It'll help you feel absolutely fantastic and will support everything else that you've been doing in this program so I want you to go through it and systematically remove everything negative from your life. Here's why. Why not?

What negative thing do you have in your life that's making your life better. I can't think of any. If you find one, call me and write to me. I'd love to hear about it but there's very few things that will ever really add to your life and help you get rid of get rid the negative people get rid of the negative TV the negative news just get rid of it and never look back and say I wish I kept it so beyond the negative people places and things. Spread your net out. Look for everything that's negative in your life and just get rid of it. OK. Just a couple of final thoughts here. Everybody, I want to remind you of something that's very important: there's no such thing as a defective baby. Look at this beautiful child here. That's you.

You were born beautiful, innocent and perfect. Your mind was fresh. There was never anything wrong with you. You're not defective. You're not bad. Life is not especially cursing you. You're beautiful, innocent and perfect. That is your natural state. When you remove all the negative thoughts, all the old programming, everything we've been trying to move you away from. And you just replace it with positive inputs coming in from life that are desperate to get inside of you. You will go back to being beautiful, innocent and perfect in such a way that you can feel it. Now this is who you are. Everything else is simply rubbish covering it up that simply needs to be cleared away. There is nothing wrong with you, you're beautiful so be gentle and give yourself the time you need to heal.

Healing is a process that doesn't happen in a day, it doesn't have to take years either. I've seen people do total transformations in just a matter of weeks or months. It goes very quickly. Why? Because once you start focusing on the right things once you have the right tools. Once you know what to do and now you know what to do. Once you start taking action. Start working for yourself instead of against yourself. You heal very quickly but take a little bit of time each day to work on yourself and a little bit of time just to rest. Reflect, heal , let your mind relax, let your mind go blank. Give yourself the freedom to heal much as if you were ill you would take some time to rest. I want you to rest your mind a little bit every day.

Let me leave you with this thought. Being a good person is the only success you need. And remember you were born beautiful, perfect and innocent. You are a good person. There's nothing wrong with you, you're beautiful, innocent and perfect and it was just covered up. There might have been a lot of bad things that happened to you but they are not about you. They do not define you. You are a good person and that's what defines you. You are already a massive success in life.

Think of it this way if you know a butthead a real jerk and they've got the trophy spouse and they've got millions of dollars and they live in the penthouse and they're driving a hundred thousand dollar car around and they've got their 10 million dollar boat and they go off in their private jet and they fly all around the world and they seem like they have average day do you like that person do you think they're a valuable person. Because I don't, I'd rather see somebody you know broke destitute living in a crap hole that has a smile on their face and they're nice to everybody they meet. That person is far, far superior.

Look at all the Buddhist monks they would beg on the side of the road they literally didn't need anything they didn't have to have degrees they didn't have to get a certain job that they have a thing they had to eat and be a good person don't die and be a good person don't die and be a good person and then share that with other people. So to be a good person all you do is don't die. Be the good person that you are and share a little bit of your joy, a little bit of your love, a little bit your kindness with the next person and you are the biggest success you can ever be in life. This has been an amazing Book and you've learned tools, strategies and techniques to get that life second to none.

You've got more coping skills now than ninety nine point nine percent of the country will ever have. They'll go from the cradle to the grave, from the womb to the tomb and never have as many coping skills as you do now. I want to offer you this. We've got a great sister program. It will literally double the number of coping skills you have in this area to make you feel absolutely fantastic. That's why we entitled it to mental freedom, freedom from pain. So if you want to literally double your skills you want to feel absolutely fantastic. You won't have these tools for yourself, for your family or for your friends. Go ahead and google mental freedom, freedom from pain and get this wonderful companion program minus . I want to thank you for coming today. You've been absolutely fantastic.

You've been massively successful, you've done a fantastic job. I admire and respect you because you're working on yourself. That is the best thing you can be in life. Check out my other resources at my advanced ideas dot com or do a google search for and you'll find my other chapter. I hope to see my very nice chapter. I just want to share with you that I think you're absolutely fantastic. You're the person that has done the work. That's why you're here. That's why you're at the end because you're a winner. So if nobody's told you you're amazing today let me be the first and I hope to see you in my very next chapter.

Communication - Goals & Benefits

Hi everybody and welcome to the Advanced Ideas chapter on "Winning With Communication." Won't you please give a warm welcome to Professor Cline. This is my good buddy J.J here ... he's our corporate mascot. Let's start with a couple of goals. The first goal is to increase your understanding of how communication works. That's a great goal right? 2) How to Improve Your Communication. I think that's what everybody is here for. 3) We really want to improve our relationships and our impact on others. So we've got some amazing benefits for you here today. The first is to say things in such a way that others will ACTUALLY listen to you. Wouldn't that be a delightful change? Next, is to learn how to make your communication more powerful, more impactful.

We also want to improve your relationships. Communication is the foundation of relationships. We want you to be more influential, to be able to have more impact on people, to be able to convince them, to make changes, and to motivate them. We also want to help you get your needs met. That's one of the major reasons why people communicate at all. We also want to create closeness and understanding with others. I think that's a beautiful goal to have. We want you to be more liked, because we work with people and we do business with people we know, LIKE, and trust. And in our social life, It's just so much better to be liked. Next we want to understand others better, so we can understand why they do the things they do, and we can learn a lot of that, through how they communicate, and also how they miscommunicate.

You'll see that as we move forward, and ultimately the goal of this chapter is to help you achieve your goals. So, I love this graphic here, "Hear no evil, See no evil, Speak no evil." It really talks to some of the communication errors that we have, and that we'll be talking about as we go through the chapter. There's a lot of people who say something, and like in the first example, "hear no evil." They can't seem to hear what you're saying. In the second example, "See no evil." They hear what you're saying but they really can't quite picture it. They're not quite getting it. In the third example, "Speak no evil." They've had some challenges, they didn't like something you said. They want to give you some feedback but what did they do? Instead, they stay silent. So, these are the "Three Deadly Sins."

There are also some of the "Deadly Sins Of Communication," and we'll talk more about that as we move forward in the chapter. Remember, master communicators, know. Write this down. "To Listen And Understand Before They Try To Speak And Be Heard." So a lot of communication is what I call "Intelligence Gathering." I want to listen to what people are saying. I want to get an understanding of their values, their belief systems, how they picture the world,. To get a full understanding of what's going on for them, what they're talking about, the nature of the challenges that they have, and what they may or may not be open to right? Then, I'm ok to go forward, and speak, and try to be heard.

That way I can do it more impactfully, more intelligently. So, always gathering information first, and then speaking. Also, when you listen first, people feel like you're really hearing them. Well, that's on account of you are. So, it's not an optical illusion, and when people feel that they've been heard, Guess what? They're much more likely to listen to what you say. So, no matter how you calculate it, this is the best system for doing it. Now, here's a great quote. "Good communication is about creating a bridge between minds", and I just love this graphic. Absolutely beautiful, and that's what you're doing. You're trying to get one mind to communicate with another mind and to truly understand it. That's really difficult.

It's one of the things that we're going to talk about next, because speaking and actually being understood are two completely different things. Let me give you a good example of that. The telephone game is the perfect example. You give one little phrase and you let it go around the room through five or six different people and when it gets back to you, it's totally miscommunicated. I say something like Go grab me the stapler and it comes back, beat the lamp with a banana. (LOL) Now, you think that's an absurd example but that's an actual example from one time when I did this with a group.

It sounds bizarre, but little miscommunications, multiplied across multiple people, will get to become a massive miscommunication and it happens very quickly. So, here's a very simple example of how people can misconstrue what you say, and I'm only going to say four words. So, follow me through the graphic, what I said was "You look nice today".

Now, we're trying to make a very simple communication here. But look what happens when we look at the chapter with what they heard. So, my communication was, "You look nice today". What they heard was, "What, did I look like crap yesterday?" That's one way to interpret it, right?. And they are free to interpret what you say, ANY way they want.

So, here's what you say. And then, there's their interpretation of it. So, we keep trying to control the message but we also need to control the interpretation. Somebody might also say, well, you know, 's just being nice. Maybe, maybe not. Maybe that's sarcasm. Oh, you look nice today. Well, you know two can play that game, and they're going to come back at you. So, there's a lot of miscommunication even in the most simple of communications, but we're going to teach you how to beat that. So, fear not.

Key Principles Of Communication

Hey everybody, welcome back. In this chapter, we're going to talk about the key principles of communication. And the first principle you need to understand. Go ahead and take out your notebook and write this down. Is that "Communication Is The Response You Get." People say, "well, I said this a certain way and they were meant to feel loved by that and they took it wrong, so that's all on them." No. Remember, we're trying to master communication and we can't master it by blaming other people. We have to use the one tool that we have, our ability to communicate and make sure that we're getting the correct response. OK.

So, they're hearing what we're actually saying. And strangely this is one of the hardest things, we just talked about the last chapter. It's one of the hardest things in communication to actually say something and to have the other person understand it the way you said it. But, remember from the last chapter that our goal is to create a bridge between two minds, so that we're linking up, we're syncing up, and they do understand us, and that we get the response that we want for trying to make somebody happy, we want them to be happy.

We're trying to cheer somebody up, we want them to be cheered up. So, always be looking for the response that you're getting, and make sure you're getting the correct response, and that the response is what you actually think it is. So, you can see this angry couple over here and they're back to back and obviously they were communicating. They're in love.

They want to get back to the love, but the communication that they're putting out there, is it creating closeness or distance? Clearly it's creating Distance. So that's the response that they're getting. So what do they need to do? They need to change their communication. People in the middle are doing a pretty good job. They want to cheer their friend up.

Their friend is having a hard time, but she's OK with listening. She's still feeling bad. You're not going to instantly make somebody feel better just by saying something, but, see the girl's hand on her shoulder?. The friend is putting his hand on his shoulder. She's still open, she's still willing to be touched. She's still willing to communicate. The other friends were actually holding her hand on the other side. This is good communication. It will get the response that they want. That means, we love you, we care about you, we're here for you. Now, a lot of times we think we're getting a certain response back but we're not. See the person doing the OK symbol, the hand, well that means "OK" in this country.

In other countries, that's actually a response that refers to an orifice that I believe is directly located centrally between the left and the right butt cheek. And they're calling you that. That's not good communication when you're trying to present something positive, but is it good feedback? Yes, it's excellent feedback, and we will talk about that later. People are always giving you excellent feedback. The next chapter, I'm going to show you how easy it is for us to mess up our communication. So, communication is also about meaning and what we do is, we tend to assume. Look at the lady with the black eye. Did you have an immediate response to that? Did you think you understood what had happened to her? Are you pretty sure that you were right? What could this mean? The reality is, it could mean multiple things.

We don't know. But the mind, the hardest thing for the mind to do, is to put a question mark in place, to have a vacuum. Do not insert an answer immediately. Our brain's goal is to see something, evaluate it, boom, and give us instant meaning. It will do that at a high rate of speed, in like a millisecond, even when it's wrong. How many different things could this picture mean? The lady with the black eye. It could mean she's abused. And that's the common meaning. It's called a "Mental Heuristic." A heuristic is a "Mental Shortcut." I don't care if I'm right or wrong, when I can make a quick decision, I use this mental shortcut. That's what your brain does. It will go with the percentages. It says, "Boy, if I said that woman was abused or she was beaten I would be right about 80-90 percent of the time.

So, I'll go with that." Unfortunately, our brain, when it uses heuristics, also tends to stop at heuristics, it doesn't question it. It believes it and he starts telling a story behind how she got abused or how horrible this is. You know, it drives right past. Is that true or not? and starts saying, "oh my god that's horrible. And this guy beat her and he shouldn't have done that. Why wasn't she protected? Is she hurt? Does she need a hug?" You know it goes on all this stuff and it's like. Hold on, hold on, slow down. You haven't proven that this is what happened. She could have had an accident on the ski slopes. She could have banged into something, she could have had eyelid surgery, Maybe she's beautifying. Maybe she was in a fire and her eye was burned. OK. Could have been an industrial accident, this might have been a chemical burn at work.

This could be secondary to doing a scene in a movie or a horror film. This could be, she's just doing a tutorial on how to apply makeup. Matter of fact, that may be the most valid reason for why you're seeing a picture like this. You know why?, take a real close look at her eyes. What do you see? You see rings in her eyes? I know you don't know this, because why would you. But that's a classic circular ring that's lighting for photography. So likely, she's doing a demonstration of how to create makeup like this. So no, she wasn't abused, but she was trying to appear abused and she's demonstrating the makeup for you. See how quickly we jump to conclusions? But it could be a million different things. Look at the gentleman in the middle. Normally just say, "Oh, I know what's happening with him. He's tired.

It's so clear, it's right there." Have you never seen a tired person before? But, is that what it means? He could have a sleep disorder. He just falls right to sleep all the time. Could be a sleep disorder. He could be amazingly intoxicated or drunk. OK. It could mean he's bored. He's not tired. He's bored. Look at the lady screaming here over on the right. What could that mean? People would say, "I know what that means. That means she's frustrated." No. She could be screaming for joy. She might have won the publisher's clearinghouse. "Here's your $30 million." Here's your check, they show up with the BIG check, remember that? Could be she's having a cluster migraine headache, could be she's having massive tooth pain. We don't know.

But notice that the brain uses that shortcut, that heuristic, and immediately leaps on a meaning. We have this challenge and other people have it as well. Now this is huge in communication. They did this study a long time ago. They've done it over and over and over again, the percentages change a little bit, but it always comes back to about these percentages. I remember when I was a kid. I always worried about saying the wrong thing. I said communication is all about what you say because you're speaking words, hello, you're speaking words. It must be all about what you say. But when we look at the study, you look at the sciences behind communication.

They do the studies, they check things out and they look at what percent of what is what. And here's what it breaks down to. Only 7% of the entire communication, what people are hearing, what their understanding, is actually verbal. That means 93 percent of your communication has absolutely nothing to do with what you say. That's amazing. It's more how you say it and how you use your body language. Those are the big two. That's what comprises 93% of all communication. So, I didn't think this was true. I thought it was what you say and not how you say it. And my cousin Johnny, we were driving around the car. We were arguing about this back and forth. Come to find out he was right. He says, ", enough of this. I'll prove it to you." And what he does is, he goes to the tollbooth.

He gives the lady 50 cents. And he says, "Screw you very much!" And she says, "Oh thank you!" Well, he just told her to go screw herself ... But he said it in such a way with a big smile on his face and he's waving his hand to her, like he's just seen his best friend at the airport, and 93% of the communication was that he was thrilled to see her and like her best buddy. The other 7% what he said was, "Screw you very much." OK, a little negative there ... but he proved his point, because she was so happy, she misheard it. Why? Because 93% was going in one direction, 7% was going the other direction. Your brain kicks in the heuristics we just talked about and said "oh, he must be thrilled and happy with the service he got and to see me. That's great. Most people aren't that excited to see me. It's only a tollbooth and you're giving your money away.

I don't normally get a very positive response." I'm hearing what I want to hear, which is that this person is thrilled finally, so he's happy with my service. I'm taking their money and he was so happy. It was a miscommunication. But, he had a massive advantage ... He had 93% going in the direction he wanted to go. So, he proved me wrong! TONE is very important. We're going to go over that next. Tone will change the entire meaning of the message. I heard a speaker once. He gave an example, he said, "My mother would call my name and she would say " (strong tone) vs. " (soft tone). I was going to have two totally different experiences, right?" Tonality is huge. People do voice overs. Why do they do these brilliant voice overs? Now it's nice to start out with a good voice, but you can start out with a good microphone, and just mess with the voice in the background.

The people that are really good at doing voice overs have vocal variety, tonal variety. Their pitch goes up and it goes down. It adds emotion, it subtracts emotion. It's all this tonality, it's tone. They're doing amazing things with the tone. The verbal part, the text that they're given isn't going to change. So what do they have to play with? What's the only string in the guitar that they can play on? It's the tone. And they don't amazing things with it. Body Language. 55% of human communication is Body Language. Haven't you always wondered why people talk with their hands? It's hard for people to think and even to communicate, if they have to put their hands at their side. Body language is huge. Go ahead and take your TV and shut the sound off. You know what? You'll still know about 1/2 of what's going on.

You can kind of sort of figure out what's going on and follow the story even though you're essentially what? DEAF! There is no communication in terms of verbal or tone. But still get what? About 55% of it. So, remember these percentages and try to be good at your communication in these percentages. Stop worrying so much about the verbiage, what you say. Worry a little bit more about the tone and use real good strong body language to communicate the feeling. The sense of things. The true message that you want to get across. Now let me show you a little bit about the tone. It's one of the most powerful keys to effective communication. I'm gonna use an example here, and I'm going to use the exact sentence, I'm gonna use the exact same seven words over and over and over again. And all we do is change the TONE and I will totally change the meaning. Are you ready? "I" didn't say, he took the money. I "DIDN'T" say, he took the money.

I didn't "SAY", he took the money. I didn't say, "HE" took the money. I didn't say he "TOOK" the money. I didn't say he took the "MONEY". Now, I said six different ways and each one had a totally different meaning, simply based on tone. The tone that I used, the word that I keyed on. Literally the way I described the words on the screen with what, just the tone. Add in some body language, and it could be wildly different. That's it for these tips and I'll catch you in the next chapter.

We Are ALWAYS Communicating

Hey, welcome back. You're doing absolutely fantastic. So, in this chapter, we're going to teach you something that you may not have been aware of. It's that you're always communicating. We're always communicating. We can't stop communicating. We do it in a multitude of ways but we're always communicating, even when you're sitting there saying nothing. This would always drive therapy clients nuts. A lot of therapy clients thought they could just sit there and say nothing throughout an entire interview, and they would be resistant. They just sit there with their arms folded and they thought that they were telling you nothing. Oh, no, you were telling me a ton. You were telling me that you were resistant, that you didn't want to be in treatment, that you were angry, that you were upset, that this actually worked maybe on your parents, or your coworkers, or somebody who's not me.

This didn't work on me. I knew that it was a gambit, a gambit is basically a power ploy that you're trying to use, that you figure that I can't defeat. I go in and I am doing an assessment on a client, and they would just sit there and they would say nothing, but they were communicating. I could communicate back and make sure I got them to communicate. I'd say hey, it's going to be very difficult to do your intake if you don't communicate. Can you help me out, and they were very sincere in their answers. They said nothing. They were just, absolutely flat. So, I would communicate with them. I'd say, I'll tell you what. Given the fact that I can't do the intake. I've got a long line of people outside waiting for you.

I got your probation officer, who's going to do the paperwork, and I've got the police officer that he's got a set of silver bracelets, and he's going to take you in the green, and white taxi called the police car, and he's going to take you off to jail, and they've got your old orange jumpsuit. They still have one left in your size. I can see from your chart here, your name is John Michaels. OK. But good news. They still have your old number. So, instead of being John, you can go back to being 9 7 2 8 4 9. You won't even have to remember a new number. So, today's going to be a great day for you. So, I need to know if you want to come into treatment, and I need to know in the next 10 seconds or, you and I are going to part ways, and I'm going to let the next person in. The probation officer is not a patient man.

Well, I didn't say, I wasn't going to talk, you know. Can't you give a guy a minute to think, all of a sudden you get this major turnaround, but realize people are always communicating. When somebody does something, when they don't do something, when they choose to do something, when they choose not to do something, when they're being helpful, when they're being hurtful, it doesn't matter what is going on, they're always communicating, where they pay attention to you, they don't pay attention to you, they get excited about what you're saying, they don't get excited about what you're saying. People can not stop communicating. I'll bet there's a situation where you think there was no communication, but you also think there was a lot of communication.

You've got a date with a girl and you say hey, let's meet together at this restaurant at 8:00 and she doesn't show up. Is that communication? Yeah, you're thinking it is. You know, it means something. Does she hate you? Did she forget? Should I call the hospitals? I'm going to call the local hospitals and she better be in one. What does it mean? It means something. Everything is communication. Let's take a look a little deeper. Now, here's some different ways to communicate. I don't want to belabor them. First one is facial expression, that's absolutely huge, but don't be deceived by facial expressions, facial expressions are very consistent.

They're very accurate but I want you to know, nobody ever practiced their facial expressions in the mirror. The only person that's good at deceiving people with facial expressions, is liars because they actually will practice it in front of a mirror, but, honest sincere people, can also sometimes have facial expressions that don't always match up with how they're feeling. I remember when I would sit in the bus at high school and i'm finally done, I could relax for a few minutes. My work day at school is over. I'm taking the bus but then I'm going to my job, I have after school, and I'm just going to relax, and I'm like in perfect serenity and I'm just like reading the green grass whiz by, and the trees, and the clouds in the sky, and I'm just kind of drifting out, and looking out the window, and people are like, why are you so depressed, depressed is the best part of my day.

So, looking relaxed can also look depressing to another person, doesn't mean that's what you're necessarily feeling but it's what they're seeing in what they're interpreting, remember, what we said, those aren't the same things. So, the next one is hand signals. I think that's a great way to communicate. Aggression is another way to communicate. That guy just talked about, sitting there, you know, in the interview room just folding his arms. He wants to use aggression. I said, well, that's his style of communication all matched to, right? I'll use the exact same style and I'll do it. Why, because he only does this once, I've done this a million times. I'm going to have better techniques than him. I've seen a lot of customers, so aggression is a form of communication. Now these are forms of communication which are actually levels, if you do a letter or email.

I want you to hearken back to the last chapter, 7 percent of communication is what, verbal is the spoken word or what, written word. It's the text, literally. So, if you send a letter, an email, a text, they only hear the words, they only read the words, I'm sorry, they don't even hear them, they only see the words. That's 7 percent of the communication. That's terrible. That leaves 93 percent to fall on the ground into what, you got it, be misinterpreted. Telephone. Well, now you got the words that's seven. You've got the tonality. That's good. That's 38. Now you're up to what, I'm carrying the one, that's 45 percent, OK. Fifty five percent of the communication. OK. Unless you use FaceTime or something like that, it is gone, why did you lose body language?

The only time it's 100 percent, and you can still have miscommunication but at least you got 100 percent of you guys on the field you know, in this battle. It's 100 percent, in person. Words, tone, body language. You got it all going on. I remember my very first girlfriend. She went off to college and we started writing the letters and we talked on the phone once in a while, and Of course when she was here I would go visit or on the weekends we talk in person, and that's when I learned how messed up letters and telephones can be. I would send her a letter, loving caring letter blah blah blah blah blah, love you think the world of you did, and she would come back all upset or I wouldn't hear from her for a while, because she was mad about something I had said cause she took it totally the wrong way.

It was a little better on the phone. You know if I sent her a letter there's like a 90 percent chance I was going to get some kind of negative response because I'd write like a two page letter. So, somewhere in there she's going to find something to take offense to, I said wrong, quote unquote, by her definition, in my mind it sounded fine, but guilty until proven innocent. Same thing on the phone. I would be having this nice conversation on the phone but about half the time I go wrong, and I'm like, why? Oh my God, could I be any more nice, could I be any more sincere. It would go wrong.

In person, once in a while, it go wrong but I could immediately clean it up and like I said I had all my soldiers in the field, i had 100 percent of the communication there, I would probably win, OK, that was OK, but man, I almost completely stopped doing the letters and I was very careful to evaluate them. Could this possibly be taken any other way before I ever send them out. I was extra careful on the phone and I kept the conversation short and then did the bulk of my communication when I was there with her in person and that made it go much much better. So, remember this in relationships and remember this in communication with businesses. Businesses love to shoot letters, emails, texts back and forth and they think the other person understands, that is not in evidence, much better over the phone.

You won't have the same challenges that I had because there's not as much emotional stuff going on, but everybody is an emotional animal. Everybody is actually more emotional than they are intellectual and even though you say, oh, it's just business. They will have challenges over the phone and could take offense to anything. Remember, there's nothing people can't take offense to. Phone call was too long and you bored me. I'm offended. It was too short. What I'm not worth your time. I'm offended. It was just right. But why did you call me three times this week?

You only call me once this week. I'm offended, too much, too little. There's a million ways to go wrong, only one way to be perfect. So, there are lots of ways to communicate. I want to share with you some of the challenges, now a lot of times, these communications can go absolutely perfect. You my girlfriend, wonderful, no challenges but we're going to teach you complete mastery to make it as good as humanly possible. Remember, you can only control your half, right? But we're going to teach at a master's degree. So some other ways to communicate, a gift, you give a gift, give a gift, that says a lot around the holidays right? A gift is very sincere.

You only do that for people you want, like, yeah, creates reciprocity. These are all forms of communication. Touches a huge one. Kagan's couple, I think, may have met once or twice, but even a simple touch has levels of communication. I used to show it to people. You would wave to somebody, that's one level of communication, you would shake their hand, you would do the warm hand-clasp where you touch their hand, you touch their elbow, you touch their shoulder while you're doing it. You say, "To hell with a handshake", bring it in, I want to give you a hug but there's different kinds of hug, there's the large circular hug where there's a foot in between you where you say, I want to maintain my frame, you maintain your frame. We will now do the tango and you're so far away from the other person, then there's guy one where the quick pat on the bat and get out of Dodge, there's the one where you get the full body hug like you give your mom, bring it in, so, touch has a lot of different levels. Snobby. Remember, we said, when you're not communicating, you're communicating. My wife, she's Filipino.

They're very poor back in the day, like Gilligan's Island, I mean, they literally lived in the bamboo hut, they literally cleaned their clothes out on a rock with a bar of soap out in the brook. So what did they have for fun? They could listen to the radio. They didn't have a TV. Again, it was like Gilligan's Island. They could go swimming. You could go for a walk, you could talk or you could eat. So, the biggest things were talking and eating and that's what they did. And they'd love to do it together. So, my wife thought the ultimate thing you could do to somebody to really hurt them, well, she'd want to starve me to death so she decided she wouldn't talk to me, she'd snub me. We literally called it snobby. Bernadette, are you snubbing me? No response.

It's snobbing right, but I'm a therapist. I talk to people all day long, I talk to other therapists, I talk to clients, I talk to insurance providers, blah blah blah blah blah. I'm not a big talker, all evidence to the contrary because I'm teaching right now but I love to have my downtime. So after a long day of like 10-12 hours of blah blah blah blah blah, me or somebody else, I loved a perfectly good opportunity to A, shut the hell up and B have some silence. It took her about three days of doing this into our marriage before she realized I was actually digging it. This was not a consequence for me, it was a reward but snubbing is definitely a communication. Posing, this is interesting, you can take a lot of ways.

Some people are always trying to stand a certain way, look a certain way, be in the right light, it can be that kind of posing but the opposite is the way that you just hold your body, you naturally do it. Everybody is posing without realizing they're posing because it's not a fake pose it's a real pose. I stand like this, I look like this, I hold my body like this it can be anywhere from. I always look like I was walking around with a stick up my butt, people said, Why? well, I got a lot of curvature in my spine so it probably does look like I'm walking like that slightly, bowlegged. I've got an extra foot, a little bit shorter than the other, nobody's perfect. Bruce Lee had the same problem. So, great even the way I walk, the way I stood you, you stand a little bit different. It has a lot to do with personality as well, but it's also communicating. Gestures are huge.

This is the biggest part of the what, the body language right? Signs, this could be anywhere from a sign on a wall. I used to have a sign on my wall that said, "oh [REMOVED]". Ok, I was just like the one that you saw. Science can also be things you have around the room, the room, what you choose to have in the room, what you don't have in the room. You can tell about 80 percent everything you'll ever need to know about a person just by walking around their house and looking in the various rooms. Why?, because it perfectly matches who they are in everything that says something about them, good, better and different. So, signs are another way to communicate.

What are some other ways? There's literally a million different ways to communicate. I want you to take some time. I want you to reflect. Ladies, hold in the glasses. What does that mean, is that a communication. Yes. She looks smarter with the glasses. Does she do that on purpose? Because she can't see. Does she use the glasses as a prop to look smarter as she's talking? Hey, if you don't see me then I look smarter when I'm talking with him but I can also look prettier at the same time. Is that a good technique? She may be doing it consciously, she might be doing that unconsciously, see, there's a million different ways to communicate. She's communicating. Because she has her glasses, where she's fumbling around if she doesn't ever have glasses.

That means she's absent minded at least in the air of what, her glasses. People are always communicating, what she chose to wear, girlfriend shows up on a date. Clothing is a form of communication. Did she wear her sexy clothes? We're going to get to at least second base on this date outfit or does she wear something conservative, slow your whole body. I need to know you first. You could be a serial killer, stalker. OK. So, everything is saying something. I want to go out for at least the next day and see how many different ways people are communicating. I want you to think about it when you're reading a TV show, when you're doing something, when you're reading people interact, when you're in an interaction. Notice that people never,ever ,ever stop communicating.

It's your ability to pick out the sheer number of ways that they communicate to have this awareness and to begin to see it, and the only way you can do that is to practice. That's your homework for today and I'll see you in the next chapter.

Fundamentals Of Communication - Part 1

Hey, everybody welcome back. Great to have you here. In this chapter we're going to look at the seven fundamentals of communication and we'll break it down into parts because there's seven of them, a little bit lengthy. So, the ones that are going to look at today are goal oriented, strategy, process, influence, feedback adjustment in meaning. So, let's jump right in. First of all, every communication should have a goal. A lot of people forget this. They go in there and they don't even know what they want to accomplish, what they want to have happen, you know. If you've got your goal how would you know you actually got it? None of this stuff is considered. So, let's break it down.

The first thing, the absolute most important thing you need to know is, what are you trying to accomplish? Second thing is, how do you know if you're successful? Literally, how would you know if you accomplished it and finally, what do you want to have happen. So, do you want somebody to buy something, take an action, maybe not take an action. Sometimes that can be equally good, right? What do you want to have happen? What's your ultimate outcome if this was your dream scenario and everything went perfectly, what would that look like and how close or how far were you from that when you left the room. That's kind of how you'll evaluate your communication and your ability to influence the other person.

So, take good notes when jot these down or print this screen out. These are the things you should always be thinking about. You should never go into a communication that's important and try to wing it. Use this as your list. Next part, I love this, this is a strategy that's why use a chess board because it's literally talking about, what is your plan. How are you going to get from point A to point B to point C to point D, etc all the way through. Think it through, the quality of your outcome is usually based on the quality of your plan, right? Next, what strategies, what techniques are you going to use. That's very helpful to making sure that what, plan goes through, plan works, you always want to be able to support your ideas.

You don't want to communicate and go blah, blah, blah, blah, blah and hope it works. No, I know what the objections are going to be and I know how to support my ideas when they have the objections. I know I'd overcome them, salesman figures if they can go out there they've got a good product. You need the product or you wouldn't be talking, what stops the sales. It's a series of objections, so salesmen and this would be very simplistic. They basically think that if they can get over every objection, every reason that's blocking you from buying, the natural fact that you need the item will complete the sale.

They're not wrong. So, always be looking for what are the potential objections and how can I overcome them. How can I make sure that people see my ideas as rock solid and a contingency plan? There's an old expression that says, "Man makes plans and then guides laughs." I don't know if you're religious or not but it's a good expression, right? You make plans and then life laughs in your general direction. Life is defined as a series of problems. You're going to have this wonderful plan, this brilliant strategy, you think you nail down all the objections and bam, they're going to hit you with something out of the blue. It could be that the building catches on fire. I don't know. The communication gets interrupted, what do you do if you only get halfway through.

You know, do you close it? You wait? What do you do? So, contingency plans always have those in place before the meeting not after the meeting and finally for this chapter, understand that communication is a process. Think of it like a recipe and I love this cute picture, this little girl is so sweet. It's literally like baking a cake. There's certain things they have to do first, second and third. Imagine if you were baking a cake, you got all the processes right but you don't have the sequencing right. So, you take a box of Betty Crocker mix, you throw the box in the oven, you cook it to 350 degrees for 20 minutes. You pull it out, you empty it into the pan. You shove an egg and some water into it and you blend it and then you serve this to your family. Did you do all the processes correctly? Yes. Did you do the sequencing correctly? No.

So, in a communication, if you want it to go well, sometimes you go to plan these things out. What am I to say first, second and third, and the sequencing is very important. How do I build momentum? Is also sometimes important, if you're trying to make a sale or sell somebody an idea of buying something or doing the next right thing, or taking a positive action for them, or for you. You want to build momentum as you go through and finish up on your strongest point. They say those who finish big win big. So, what is your big finish? How are you going to bring it home? I like to make my strongest point last and do it with a little bit of emotion. I think that's a good formula and if you do that, you'll finish big and you'll win big. I'll see you in the next chapter.

Fundamentals Of Communication - Part 2

Hey, everybody welcome back. Now, in this chapter of looking at the seven fundamentals of communication part two. We're going to look at influence and this is a fascinating one, shameless plug. I've got an entire chapter on persuasion strategies that you absolutely love because I'll tell you, without the ability to persuade people, to motivate them, to influence them you're not going to get much done in life. So, one of the first things you want to do in communication is look at what tools of influence you're going to use, either take my Book or gather them but have a tool chest of communication skills specific to influence that you can use in any situation and then go ahead, and plug them into the important upcoming situation, and you'll do absolutely fantastic.

Now, also notice what tools they're most susceptible to you know might be appealing to their ego or vanity, or their greed, or their need to do good in the world, it can be a lot of different things that you can use and there's a million different tools like I said but everybody has certain ones that work better on them and worse on them. So, pick the best of the best. Specific to them, your target audience and match to the other key thing with influencing somebody is understanding how they see things. It doesn't matter how you see things when you want to be influential. You have to come from their place where they're at. Meet them where they are, understand how they see things and then influence things based on their version of reality because we all have our own versions of reality.

Next, always be looking for win-win situations. Not I win, you lose, you win, I lose. No no, win win situations are the absolute best. I'll tell you about at least, at least nine times out of 10. You can find a win-win situation that will allow you to influence the person. You can feel great about it. They can feel great about it. We call that what everybody wins. Next is feedback. So, look at what kind of response you're getting. Are they happy? Are they concerned? Are they upset? Are they taking it in? Are they accepting it? Are they rejecting it? Do they look like they have questions in their mind? Always be scanning, scanning. What are you hearing? What do you see almost in you know, from a gestural perspective. What are you feeling? What's coming back from this person?

People I communicate best are best at sensing what's going on. What type of response are they getting from the other person then their response is almost obvious. It's a reply to what they're sensing from the other person, that makes it easy if you don't have that, it's very difficult, i don't care how skilled you are, so focus as much on what the other person is giving you back as in what you're going to say. Most people try to figure out boys. I hope I present well. I do this or that. They're worried about their chapter and not about the feedback from the other person. That is a mistake. The next most important thing to consider is what are their concerns, what are their objections. Remember, if we can get past these, we what? That's right. We make the sale.

So, always be looking, see are they pleased or are we getting a positive response and always keep checking to make sure that you're understood. and a lot of people say, "Hey you understand the goal." Oh yeah. No, they don't. You have to check and look at all the signals that they're giving you to make sure that they understand. Sometimes I'll ask somebody to do something as simple as repeat it back to me or I'll ask them a clarifying question: if you were to get your perfect outcome, what would it look like? and they start talking about something that was nothing that I was talking about. and I realized that they didn't understand even though they very sincerely shook their heads. Yeah, oh yeah I understand what I understand. No, they understood the question.

They thought I was asking and not the question I actually asked. So, when you ask him, do you understand, a lot of times they look very sincere like they do understand it and yes they do understand, they understand their wrong interpretation of what you said and you look at them and say, Oh they're very sincere. I can see they clearly understand just by looking at their faces. Now, you've got to get them to engage in the conversations in some way shape or form such as to show you that they actually understand then you've got to win. Now, communication like most things in life is all about adjustment, so be looking and thinking to yourself kind of go down through this as your checklist. Do I need to change my strategy? Try to do a little more of this, a little less of this. Maybe I need a whole rethink.

Maybe I should switch strategies. What tools, strategies, techniques in my use that are currently getting the best responses, maybe I want to use more like that, stand that thread. Always be looking at where there's resistance. You know, how can I cut down resistance, how can I overcome resistance. How can I go around resistance, so I don't have it in the first place? Be a little proactive and adjust to what's going on in the other person in terms of body language, tone and positioning. You want to see what's going on for the other person. The last chapter I told you will be listening, listening, listening which means scanning, listening to their body language, listening to their tone and the positioning. You want to make sure that you adjust for these things. This is the feedback that you're getting. So, the last chapter was, am I listening to the feedback, am I making the adjustments to the feedback.

Is this chapter? Finally meaning, are they getting the right message not just any message the correct message. That's the hardest thing to get across. So, focus on them, get that feedback, make sure they're getting the right message. Lots of people want to take things the wrong way. You've got to massage them a little bit, romance a little bit. Turn them around. Get them moving in the right direction. Notice some of the things that you're doing that are helpful or hurtful. Should I use a little more emotion, a little less emotion. What's the right amount? How is my tone impacting the meeting? The meeting. So, you want to look at how your words are impacting it. Your tone is impacting it and next, body language.

So, we're always really concerned with how what I'm saying, how that's going over but again remember, tone and body language are 38 percent and 55 percent for a total of 93 percent of the communication and the meaning that they're getting from the communication. We did some demonstrations, how important these things are. Make sure you're looking at those things as you're going through this important communication. A lot of times I noticed that a simple change of something is kind of obscure as pace. Was I talking too fast? Was I talking too slow? Should I have slowed down on certain words, ok. That's pacing, slowing down at certain points. We call them sometimes pregnant, pauses are important. So pacing can be very important. That's it for this chapter. You're doing absolutely fantastic. And I'll see you in the next chapter.

Great Communication Tips - Part 1

Hey everybody, welcome back. Now we're going to go over some great Communication Tips And here's your very first one and this is kind of an overriding one that you want to be looking at constantly as you're presenting which is what communication is when you're presenting to somebody you want to look at. Is it helping or is it hurting. Think of it this way. I'm trying to make a sale. Is it getting me closer to closing the sale or farther away. I want to connect with somebody by creating a connection or disconnection. I want to keep people interested. Is it creating interest or lack of interest like this poor guy nose down on the table noticing which one you're doing by getting this feedback. This will help you stay on track. Hit the right spot and actually move in the direction you're trying to move it.

Great great tip. Now here's a little piece of reality. People are much more interested in Hello and much more interested in what they have to say than what you have to say. People are always going to be more excited about talking in a conversation than listening in a conversation. We're going to talk a little bit later on about conversational generosity and how that works. And this will make more and more sense to you as you go on. But a lot of people think conversation is about being a great talker. A lot of times it's about being a great listener and being as interested. Sometimes if you want to create excitement of being more interested in what the other person has to say than what they're saying that will create high likeability with the person, help you connect with them and ultimately make the sale area trying to sell someone an idea, a product , a concept , maybe even helping themselves.

Let's dive a little deeper into this. Most people actually aren't communicating, they're just taking turns talking. People are literally waiting for you to take a breath so they can jump in and say the next brilliant thing that they thought of. Here's our typical conversation: you say something that sparks an idea in the person that you're talking to. They start subvocalizing internal self-talk and they go blah blah blah blah blah. What they thought about your very first idea. Now everything you say after the first idea they pretty much missed. Then they get to talk and they say this is great. I mean tell this person something and you're going to get all this information. Then they say something. And the first thing that they say triggers something in you.

You start thinking about it and you're saying blah blah blah blah blah in the back of your mind thinking about how brilliant you are about going over what they had just said and you miss the next 15 things that they say because you're talking in your own head. And this cycle repeats and repeats and repeats. So what we want to do is make sure that when we're talking with somebody we're getting good communication across. And one way that you can do that is to interrupt them with a question and ask them a question about what you're talking about that will get them out of their head and focus back on what you're talking about. So

I'll say you know hey there was one time when I was in such and such a situation blah blah blah blah blah. And I'll say "Have you ever been in a situation like that?" And I give a quick minute to respond but it stops the talking in their head. And then I go on to my next point.

What I really want to tell you about is blah blah blah blah blah. Is that something that you feel you could use? The other question stops the self-talk. Whatever blah blah blah blah blah. They were doing it in their mind. They had to stop and focus and answer the question. So make sure that when you're talking to somebody that they're actually listening they're not glazed over. And when they're talking I want you to actually listen to what they're saying, not go with this subvocalization talk in your own mind. Does that make sense? Listen to what they say. You can think about it for days after. Don't spend too much time thinking about why they're talking about it except to analyze what are their values, what are their beliefs and what's important to them.

That's all this vocalization you should be doing now when you're generous in letting somebody talk almost talk themselves out and then they're more likely to listen to you and not be so hyper to jump in and when you take a breath and say something more about that later this is an interesting one. I always tell people that they are tuned into a radio station called WIfe them What's in it for me? People always want to know when you communicate. The thing that they care about the most is what's in it for them. Everybody is self motivated. That means they're motivated by what's in it for them. So when you're talking about things, don't talk about why it's important to the government or society or the world as a whole. How are they going to make money? How are they going to benefit from this? How is this going to solve their problems? How is it going to make them look good? That's all they care about.

So make sure when you're trying to get a point across that you're telling them what's in it for them. If you're not talking about what's in it for them because remember they're tuned to a radio station called WIIFM What's In It For Me. If you're not tuned into that they will tune you out. Now here's a great tip. Whenever you're networking, whenever you're talking, whenever you try to communicate with another person and you really want to connect with them. Write this down, print out the chapter whenever you need to do. It's much better to be interested than interesting. A lot of people think well of being a great communicator. To make an impression on people like you you've got to be you know funny and charismatic and say that people are starved. I can tell you as a therapist they'll pay me $300 an hour to sit there and listen to them Why.

Because they are starving for somebody to listen to them. So much better to be interested in the other person personally who cares about their concerns. What's interesting to them is that you will seem like a brilliant conversationalist if you're a really good listener. So you want to talk about half as much as you speak. They say that's why you got two ears and one mouth so that you can keep your conversation and that proportion listens twice as much as you talk. Be interested in them and find what they're saying. Fascinating. And then they will do what the LA press reciprocity says they will listen to when you speak so listening here's some main listening skills. One listen never ever misses a perfectly good opportunity to listen. Caring. Be there for that person and just be there for him, not just be listening but show them that you care. You know you say that must be so hard for you. That must have been great when that happened. Wow what was that like?

Reflect that you're actually caring, that you're interested and that you care for them. Our best friends are the ones that care for us and when our best friends talk we listen. Why? Because they care about us. Following up following you know listening is more than just you know sitting there not talking. You have to make sure that you're engaged, use eye contact, non-intrusive gestures nodding your head saying OK, asking very infrequent questions. Adding to that is so true. I remember one time when I. OK but make it very brief. That really worked for me one time. Boom you're out you're in you're out. I know that to be a true man you speak and you speak the truth to me. I know what that's like. OK. That shows that you're following.

I remember when that happened to me one time. That's the following. But in and out quickly don't get into a story that they got to listen to about you reflecting his paraphrasing and reflecting back the feelings you're sensing. Wow that must have been really hard for you. I can remember when that happened to me one time and it was really painful. Paraphrasing is saying the same thing back say no when my girlfriend left me I was absolutely crushed. Say wow I can see why you were crushed. That's paraphrasing. I can see why you were crushed. Bill: That must have been very painful for you. Painful. Another way to say crushed.

OK. So therapists are really good at this but the average person needs to get really good at this as well. And it's the final piece just for this little chapter here and great tips. This is huge. If you learn nothing else in this chapter about conversation except this conversational generosity is one of the big tips that you want to remember. Now remember because people are tuned to that radio station WIIFM What's In It For Me. When you talk this is like Einstein's theory of relativity he said you know when you spend a minute an hour with a girl it seems shorter than any minute. That's relativity right. You know and he spent an hour with a pretty girl. It seems like a minute when you spend a minute doing something you don't like. It seems like an hour. That's relativity.

So when you're talking it seems like a long time to the person when they're talking it seems like the time when his bike has a short period of time. So these percentages are pretty accurate when you talk half the time they are going to think that you took up pretty much you know two thirds to three quarters of the conversation is going to feel like 70 percent. When you talk 40 percent of the time you're going to think you were generous but it really sounds more like 50/50 to them. That's the way it feels and that's the way they remember their perception of the conversation is everything. Because this is what this is the person you're trying to talk to the person you're trying to influence their perception not reality is what is key.

So this is why I say listen twice as much as you talk because if you're talking in those proportions you're only talking about 30 percent of the time that's going to seem like about 40 percent of the time to them which is going to be noticeably less than half but just barely. So they're going to say hey this person didn't dominate the conversation. They actually listened to me. They didn't try to overpower me which means what. Talking 50/50 like everybody else you know or God help them if they ever do run into somebody you talk to 70 percent of the time they're going to feel like it was a hundred or 110 percent of the time. See how this works. I like to talk around 30 to 20 percent of the time.

And if I'm talking 30 percent of the time even part of that is going back to confirming noticing their feelings reaffirming you know they're correct in certain things where they are correct. You know, giving them validation, not just me talking about what I want to talk about. So that will seem like I'm not even talking because when you're validating somebody it seems like they're talking except they're finally getting the validation they never had before. People are starved for two things. Time to talk and validate. Those are the two things that they are craving and they are starved for so remember that and communication.

So depending upon how much you want people to like you I would say never do more than 40 percent. You want to live in that 30 percent and down category. And the more you want them to like you go down down down down down. If I really want somebody like me I go to 10 to 20 percent. I hardly ever talk and I spent half that time validating, confirming , and rephrasing, letting them know that I'm connecting and letting them know that I'm emotionally attached to what they're saying. So I'm really even if I'm talking 20 percent of the time I'm really only saying something 10 percent of the time. The rest is to support them. Same thing with the 10 percent I'm really only talking about 5 percent one twentieth of the conversation.

The other 5 percent is validating them. So go ahead and really drop down your numbers, start to listen way more than you talk, start to do the validation, paraphrasing everything that we talked about. And if you just follow the tips in this one chapter you will do significantly better and you will be a true master of communication. But don't worry we've got more and I'll see you in the next chapter.

Great Communication Tips - Part 2

Hey everybody, welcome back. You're now in the seventh chapter and we're going to do more great Communication Tips. But I want to congratulate you. You are more than halfway done and you have learned a ton of information. You are not the same person that started this chapter. Why? Because you have so much more skill and so much more mastery. Much more to come. Let's jump into this next chapter. It's absolutely amazing. Now your next tip is that the person who asked the question controls the conversation. This is amazing. You can control any conversation by simply asking a question.

Even if you're nobody. I remember when I was in high school a friend of mine taught me this skill. I said to my buddy Nick I said Man my classes are so boring. The teacher never talks about any good stuff that I want to hear about. You know and he said a simple thing to me. Did you ask any questions in class? I know a teacher knows me. I just sit there and shut up. He said no no no no no. The teacher actually works for you. And here I control him like a puppet on marionette strings. So here's what you do. Simply ask a question. They're so excited that somebody is actually interested in their class they're going to go ahead and answer the question. They can't not answer the question.

They're going to be thrilled to answer the question and guess who's controlling the conversation now no longer them. But if you don't interrupt them that teacher will do whatever they had planned for that day or whatever floats into their head that will be the entire conversation but with one simple question. Boom you can completely change the direction of the conversation as long as it matches up even slightly with what they're talking about even if it's even remotely on target. If you can even kind of force it in the shoe box it is in. So it's remotely on target or on topic. They will be thrilled to answer that question. Well I tried this out in high school a few times and I would ask some even some pretty obscure questions.

But the teacher was always more than good about answering the question in the kind of excitement that I even asked. So this technique absolutely worked. When I went out into the work field what I could do is I could change the conversation by simply asking a different question. I learned later in psychology that this is actually a powerful drive of the mind. If you think about the mind, what does the mind actually do? It asks and answers questions about what this means. And then it gives an answer. What should I do about this? And it develops a what answer when you're talking in a conversation you're largely asking and answering questions.

It's not the only thing you do but it's a huge component right. But people don't realize that you can control the conversation directed at it. Because once I ask you a question your brain is literally compelled. Compelled to answer that question. Very hard to get around it. Now having realized this I'm hoping this will help you stay on track. When people ask you odd questions that throw you off track, what you do is you learn to loop back around. You kind of answer their questions and make it relate back to what you were saying originally and then go back on with what you were saying. So that's how to get around this because I don't want you to get trapped by this either. Now let's dig a little bit more into how questions can control the conversation. So questions can do an awful lot of things.

Questions can impact mood so if I say hey what's really great in your life right now you'll start thinking about all these great times that you've had in your life and things are going really well now and I can literally see your mood increase if I say what really stinks about your life right now. You'll think about all the bad things that happened and you know things that didn't happen or should have happened or how far behind you are and blah blah blah and your mood will drop noticeably. So I can impact your mood boom like that by simply asking a different question. I can ask a question like it's kind of a question.

It's almost like a statement. Don't you always succeed when you do this? You know my experience is that you always succeed. Isn't that right? So I'm making a statement. My experience, you always succeed. Isn't that right? And if it's true then what you are going to do is you to turn them around for maybe doubting themselves to feel self-confident that's an impact on their mood by asking the right question. And I pre assumed the answer. My experience is that you always succeed. Then I ask a question: what's the brain going to lock onto for the answer. What I just said isn't that true.

Well what's lasting is the brain hurt in 's experience you always succeed.

You want me to be right. You're already thinking about the times you've succeeded because the first thing that happened when I said you always succeed. Your brain said "Is that true?" And I started focusing on it. So really different psychological ways I got your brain to focus on you succeeding. Now questions can get more info. That's the common reason we think we use questions. I'm going to leave that flat right there why. Because we kind of know that that's what we do. Hey, how do you do this? Fix this, solve this, you know, complete this boom boom boom boom. We know we ask questions to get information but I want you to use clever ways to impact mood and the next one to create insights. Have you ever considered a boom of ego?

That can create insight. People say they like therapy , they'll say oh my god I'm such a loser and blah blah blah blah. I say that is true. You're still here. You're actually kind of tougher than me. You've survived everything that's ever happened to you. Some of those things I heard in the group snapped me like a twig. You know I haven't had a hard life like you so I'm not hardened. It would have crushed me. Are you sure you're a weak person? Are you or are you a strong person who's just taken a heavy beating. Year after year after year. Is that weakness or is that strength? See I'm using questions over and over and over again almost in rapid succession to give them a new insight.

They think they're weak and I think I'm actually showing them that the very reason they think they're weak they're actually strong and how I do it. I did it through a series of questions pretty cleverly right. You can do things like this all the time. When people question their courage I make them question their lack of courage when they question their strength. I make them question their lack of strength. I go in the opposite direction. I can always check my attention. So I can ask a question like when's one time that that happened to you. Have you had a similar situation? Give me an example of one time when you blink. Now somebody wasn't paying attention. I used to be able to get attention in groups and in cloud crowds simply by looking at somebody or walking around the room and I tap them on the shoulder or I would ask them a question and boom they perked right back up. It was a way to scan the crowd and to check on and garner fresh attention.

I literally was rejuvenating their attention with a nice technique right now. You can also use questions to create doubt. What's a good example of that? Well similar to the last one I gave you. Are you really a loser? Losers quit, losers don't try to get better. Losers don't come into treatment. Losers don't go to AA, they're out the bars. You literally can't be in this room and be a loser. You know my question because you don't lose until you quit. See question asked and answered. I quit. Created doubt about their weakness. You can create doubt about anything. They want somebody to think their girlfriend was cheating on them. I say I could have sworn I saw your girlfriend at the mall with somebody like a question mark. Is that going to create doubt? Yeah. Now please don't use this for evil.

But if you want to create doubt in somebody sometimes you can question it. They're telling you about the great business plan. I say how do you absolutely positively know you're going to succeed in that and they're going to come up with answers but the answers are going to be a little bit weak. Absolutely sure. See you can create weakness in creating doubt doubts will unglue ideas Attucks would tell me all my using friends promised me they wouldn't use in front of me. They promised you I would just leave the question hanging. These people are reliable. They were not they were not faithful to their word. He lent them money and they didn't give it back. You ever asked them to be someplace and they weren't there for you.

Now I'm creating doubt creating doubt creating doubt because I already know that they've lent them money and they didn't get it back. I already know these people have let them down. There are other addicts Of course he lets people down, that's what addicts do. Ok that's why the treatment. That's why they hit a bottom because they let people down. I created doubt. OK. Because I want to talk him out of a stupid idea. That's going to get them hurt. So I create doubt which loosens it up which makes it easier to defeat questions that you ask and also sets the tone. If you wanted to create the best life possible, how would you do it?

Was the tone that I just said that your life's going to be great and that there's ways to make that happen and that you can think of ways to make it happen right now. Is that moving you in a positive direction or negative direction? It's setting the tone. It's also setting what we're going to talk about right. So it's setting a topic like we talked about in the last chapter. Now I can also discover what's most important for you or why that is important to you. Uncover beliefs. Why do you think that or what would I have to believe to believe this. You know what I think to believe this. You can ask questions about the beliefs. Why is that important to you? What makes you think that's true? When did you first start believing that I can ask questions that will uncover beliefs like I say what's most important to you in life?

And they'll start telling you their values and beliefs. Great way to uncover it. What's most important to you in this deal? And by the answer that they give me under that is a value and a belief I can use questions even to interrupt patterns. Hey you know the bucks are coming to the stadium this weekend. Has nothing to do with what we're talking about. But if they were agitated, if they were upset, if they were confused, if they were hurt, it makes them think about something else which de-escalates their current state because it was interrupted. And now they have to go back to it and go oh I'm sorry you were talking about and their state has dropped whatever it was good bad or indifferent it will drop because I did a pattern interrupt and you can do that a lot of different ways. But whenever somebody states that you are getting too much of something that you don't want it to, you can just talk about anything else, just move the conversation a little bit and then go back.

It can be a stupid thing to start tapping on your phone and saying "Do you ever have a time where you know you push the power button and the thing actually shuts off?" Now that has nothing to do with what you're talking about. But it makes me think about that. It totally gets them off what they were thinking about that was upsetting them or whatever. And when they come back to what they're not as upset as they were. And you go like oh I'm sorry you were talking about and you want to go back to what they were talking about but now they're at a lower level. We used to use this in therapy a lot to de-escalate people. So questions can be very very powerful and they can do an awful lot of different things. Now here's some interesting concepts when you're talking about communication. The Greeks used to use these three concepts ethos pathos and logos ethos as ethics and character.

You always want to do things that show ethics and character. You always want to go to the Higher Self both within presenting who you are. And in describing who the other person is and people will love you for this if you describe them as having greater ethics and greater character than they actually have they will love you. The next one is pathos, passion , emotion. If you add emotion into your chapter feeling into what you're talking about with people or about people that will increase your communication in logos is just adding logic in LA times I'll say something that's very passionate and emotional a lot of personnel say but you know I know that's true because there was this one time when I saw you doing this and I was touched. I thought it was really smart when you did blah blah blah blah blah. So not only am I saying hey you're a great person I'm supporting it with facts because if you say hey you're a great person say you just saying that or you're my therapist or you're my friend or whatever or you're just trying to make a sale when I can show proof.

That my emotion, my passion behind why I feel that way about you that I do is also not so much passion but fact it's true it's real then it becomes powerful. It becomes unavoidable. Like when I tell anybody in therapy that they're a great person. Like I said Hey you're not a loser you know why. And I was reaching out to them emotionally. I wanted them to let them know that I support them. That was the pathos the logic is. Losers don't come to these meetings. Losers don't try to help themselves. This is logic. Losers aren't working out how to become a better person. Losers don't even feel bad about being losers. And that person is like that was a really nice thing to say. And that was also really true. If you just say hey you're not a bad guy that's going to roll off him like water off a duck. They'll appreciate it but they won't believe it because it's not passion backed by logic that makes sense.

And remember the ethos because that's not small either. If you are not an honest witness, if you are not using ethics and character, if you're just out there blowing smoke up everybody's crevices. They are not going to believe you. Why? Because you have no credibility. That's why I like to say you're doing a marketing webinar. When the first thing they'll always do is do the why should you listen to me part.

Why should you listen to me because I've already done what you need to do and I've got the right credentials after my name to be the person to be able to help you. I'm a good solid person and here's why I'll even talk about what path shows passion and commitment to helping you. Which one goes back to my character?

I'm the type of person that wants to help. That's a person we trust. Now last tip for this chapter: let people know that you like a lot of times you actually like something somebody. But look at these two pictures. You forgot to tell your face. Isn't that funny. You forgot to tell your face. You're not smiling. OK. Your motion is too flat. And remember we said 55 percent of communication is body language so letting people know that you liked them is a lot of different things. So look at these two pictures. Happy to see you are so happy to see you. You know one question if they're even happy to see you, the other one you know they're thrilled to see you. You can do this in a lot of ways. I'll tell people right out Hey it's great to see you. Oh my god When's the last time I actually saw you? I'm so glad we finally got together to do the handshake.

You do the hug, you do the smile, you do the warm greeting, they knock on the door and you run over any answer right away. You know you want to connect with people. There's an old expression that says the head never hears until a heart is listening. You've got to make sure that you have that heart to heart connection with somebody somebody knows that you like. We only connect with people that we know like and trust. We like people who have the common sense to like us. So you always have to let people know that you like them. This is absolutely huge in connecting and creating rapport until you have a rapport, a connection , remember that bridge of the minds that's what rapport is. No communication really happens, at least no communication that's effective. So that's your last tip for this chapter. You're more than halfway through. I am so proud of you. And I will see you in the next chapter.

Self-Talk & Powerful Language

Hey, everybody. Welcome back. We've been talking an awful lot about communication and it's always been about the other person. The other person. The other person. Now, I want to flip it on its head a little bit and talk about communication between you and you. That's right. Just me, myself and I, just the three of us. How do you talk to yourself? In therapy, we call this self talk. Sometimes it's called the inner critic. Why? Because it tends to be very, very negative. But pretty much I call it self-talk. Self-Talk is a philosophy, a system, a theory. It comes from rational, emotive behavioral therapy, also known as r, e, b t, which was started by Albert Ellis. I've actually got a nice chapter on this, if you want to check that out later.

But RB Beat is the science of how your brain works and one of the first things they teach you about is self-talk. How you talk to yourself will determine how you feel because your thoughts create your feelings, create your actions. That's the primary core of our beat. So be very careful what you think, which is self-talk, because it's going to create feelings. So when you think depressive thoughts, you think you have depressed feelings. When you think happy thoughts, you have happy feelings. So you have to be very careful.

We're not careful with our internal language, the way in which we communicate to ourselves internally, which is our thoughts, our communication with ourselves. So our communication can be empowering or disempowering. It can be discouraging or creating. Courage can either be creating assertiveness or non assertiveness. We have to be very careful how we communicate with ourselves. So I recommend our Book. There's also another Book called an NLP and it talks about language. Why? Because NLP literally stands for Neuro, which is brain linguistics, which is language and programming, how we program our brain through the use of our language. And one of the things that they teach in there I have, Of course, on this as well, is that language sets intensity.

So if you look at the scale here, it goes from peeved all the way up to furious if you tell yourself you're peeved. I put that word in there because it kind of makes me laugh all the way up to furious, like, I can't take this anymore. I'm going to explode. That language will determine how you feel. Matter of fact, I used to use this system to de-escalate people when I was a therapist. You know, when I would go in to work and, you know, they called me in on my beeper back in the day. Right. And they said, hey, you know, somebody's tearing up the game room. I go in there and I talk to the guy and he'd say, I'm furious because blah, blah, blah, blah, blah, blah, blah, Why not? And I'd say, okay, yeah, I'd be furious too, if that happened to me. You know, I'd be very mad about that.

So what I just did, I switched furious to mad very subtly. Always go one step at a time. He'd say, You're—right I'm mad. They did blah, blah, blah, blah, blah. Yeah. I can see why you would be mad. I might be upset for days. See what I did again. Mad to upset. Is there a—right I'm mad, blah, blah, blah, blah. You know, you just keep going down, down,

down through the scale. You need to do this to yourself When you tell yourself you're furious, maybe not really furious. You're mad. Maybe you need to change the language a little bit. When you get to a point where you can figure out that, Hey, I'm mad about this, you might want to say, Well, I'm really upset about this. By the time I get too upset, I can usually solve the problem when I'm mad or when I'm furious. It's hard to solve the problem.

So see how language will not only set the intensity, it will set what you can and cannot do. Resources you can access or cannot access. Let me show you that in the next chapter, a little bit more NLP for you. So we need to change the language in the top chapter. Furious, mad, upset. We talked about that. Let's go to the second chapter. Unbearable. When something is unbearable, can you bear it? Hello? No, it's unbearable. The UN can't be bearable, can't be beared. But when something's hard. Can you? It's something that's hard. Unbearable. No, it's bearable. So you can do it. It's going to be hard. It's going to be very, very difficult. But you can do it. Same thing when you use the word impossible. It's not possible. Impossible.

Can't be done. Can you solve something that's impossible? No. But can you solve something that's difficult? Yes. See how through the language your brain is using, it is physically shutting itself down. You won't intend to get out of something that's unbearable. You won't try to do something that's impossible. Impossible. When something's a catastrophe, you just sit in it. You give up. But when a catastrophe becomes a unique situation, then you can deal with it. So changing the language is absolutely huge in terms of freeing up your brain, freeing up the access to the resources in your brain. Now you can even do some reframes. Reframes and therapy are things that you say I'm a little different way.

They look different literally, as if you change the frame on a picture. You can have an average looking picture, but you can put in a good looking frame and it looks so much better. You can also take a good looking picture and put in a crappy frame and it looks so much worse. Women know this is why they change their outfits. It's the way that they frame themselves. They frame their body to make it look at its best. Guys, just go, Yeah, this is clean. I'll pop this on. Okay, So look at the bottom chapter. Problem becomes a challenge. Good use of words. Why? Because they mean the exact same thing. You've got something that you've got to fix. What do you call that? You can call that a problem. You call it a challenge. People hate problems.

The word is negative and they run away from problems. We like challenges. Challenges are fun. You play a football game against another team. Why? Because they challenged you. It's a challenge. That's what makes it fun. We like to play board games because they're challenging. We like to do puzzles because they're challenging. We love a good challenge. Matter of fact, if there's no challenge, why bother to do it? And they say, Why climb the top of Mount Everest? Because it's there. No, Because it challenges you. If it was there, but it was flat, nobody would do it. Or if it was downhill all the way. Say, man, you got to try this. It's like, you know, 6000 feet downhill. No. So change the language from problem to challenge, from failure to feedback.

This one has, you know, just like the other one has the benefit of being true. Are you a failure if you had something that didn't work out? Do you describe it as a failure or feedback? The reality of the situation. The science of the situation is you just found out one more way that doesn't work. You know, Edison had to try over 10,000 times to invent the electric light bulb. So he just said each quote unquote, failure is just part of the scientific method. Fail, fail, fail, fail, fail, succeed. Woohoo! Now you're a hero. So that's we got the motto of if you want to double your success rate, you got double your failure rate in business from science, science new. You try something. You try something.

You try something. You just keep going until you get the right solution. And you only worry not about how many times you failed, but the fact that you got the solution. That's what everybody cheers about. And it's okay. It's part of the process. I remember there was a TV show on Guy, this was way back in like the late seventies and it was about millionaires that were under the age of 35. And on average they had failed six times. So some got it in the second or third or fourth try. Other ones took ten, 15, 20 tries, but on average it was about six, six and one half failures to become massively successful. And they all said the same thing, even though they all went bankrupt multiple times, they did not care because they only needed one success.

And once they got that, they could take it to its logical conclusion. Nobody remembers the bankruptcies except it just creates a nice rocky story from rags to riches and boom, off you go. Because once you figure out the solution, you can scale it, you can multiply it, and boom, you're a huge winner. That's how Bill Gates became a big winner. He wrote a little piece of code. It became Das disk operating system way back in the day so that the computer could run that he actually did. He never did anything else. Windows Program. That was actually something that he bought from a think tank that had been working on that and had that sitting up on the shelf for like 4 to 6 years. And they never thought it would be big. They never thought it would go anywhere.

They never thought it would do anything. And he just bought it from him for like pennies. I forget what he paid, maybe ten or $20,000 or something for that. And they said, Take it, you know. And he built his multibillion dollar wealth out of that, and he never tried to do anything else. Just scale, scale, scale, scale, scale. You know, Bill Gates will tell you, I just hired people that were smarter than me to work for the company, to work the system to make Microsoft better and better and better. He didn't try to create 20 more businesses. He had the one that worked and he scaled it. Boom, you're done. Cash me out. So you can do this. It's feedback, not failure. And I'm a loser. I love that one. You're not a loser. Losers quit. If you haven't quit, you just got one more setback. Again, it's like the Rocky story. Get up one more time and you fall down. So keep going. Keep going, keep going.

Remember, you only need one success, and everybody will call you a winner. Have one or two losses. Roll over and ask people to scratch your belly and be a loser and quit. Then, yeah, you're right. But it's a self-fulfilling prophecy. You're a winner. Keep going. Don't quit. Make it happen when you find your success. Blow it up. That's the thought that I'll leave you with. And I'll see you in the next chapter.

Miscommunication

In this chapter I'm going to teach you something that you probably already know is that many times we get our signals mixed up. Go ahead and look over this cartoon. I absolutely love this one. It's a symphony to how we mess up communication. How do we do it? A lot of times it's true the power of assumptions. We assume one thing with something else is happening. We all know what assumptions actually stand for. And that's pretty accurate. We don't want to guess. Remember I talked about reflecting and clarifying and those types of things. What happens is that our communication just isn't that clear. So the question to ask yourself is is your communication clear. Here's a second question to ask yourself: Are you sure? Because a lot of times you're not as clear as you think.

Most of the time you're not as clear as you think. People will tell you if you confuse them when sometimes other times they don't. So you could confuse somebody. Say 20 percent of the time and maybe one in a hundred times they tell you the other 19 times they don't. That's 19 times that you confuse somebody and they just let it chapter. They told you about 10 percent of the number of times that you confuse them or less. And that's about the average somewhere between five to 10 percent of the time they'll tell you when you confuse them you go ha or watt or they'll let you know where they'll clean. Other times they just let it chapter by. It gives us the false illusion that our communication is clear.

There's other times where you said one thing and they heard something else like in that cartoon we just looked at and they're fine because they think they got the message. They think it was very clear. But it wasn't it wasn't the message you wanted to get across. So they got a message just not the correct message. I love this one. I used to do this as kind of a demonstration with people to show them how bad their communications were. It was called the talking feather. It was a way to do therapy in a couple of therapy to show them how bad the communication was and to remove any arguments.

So literally we had this as an old Indian tradition where you know you would sit around the circle and you would have the talking feather. It was their way to keep people from talking over each other. Great for therapists right. So they would go around the circle with the feather and whoever held the feather could talk then they could pass it around the circle or if everybody had spoken in the circle then they could pass it to somebody that raise their hand or they wanted to get a response from where they want to have shared next or get some feedback from. So that's the talking feather. Well we did the same thing in therapy. I would say give the wife the talking feather.

And then we would test to see if the husband could actually hear her. So she would talk about something I say time you got about 30 seconds and you know I'll kind of raise my hand at different levels so you know when you get towards the end kind of like when you do a chapter of like say Toastmasters and you see the yellow light the green light.

And then Of course the red light and you're out of time. So they let you know when you run out of time. So I would give her 30 seconds to talk and then she would hand the feather over to the husband and he would repeat back. You know that the core essence of what she said is that you don't have to repeat it back verbatim but just say what she was trying to tell you.

And on average these couples had to go back and forth. These are couples that have been together for many many years typically thought they complete each other's sentences and on average it took about six times to get it right. So literally we'd have to have the husband hand back that feather five more times to the wife before he could get it. Correctly. Thirty seconds of her conversation. It showed him how bad the communication was and let me tell you a second secret. The wife didn't do any better. And women are pretty good listeners. OK. They didn't do much better. You know they average like 5.5 times we just tend.

Like I said in an earlier chapter not to listen so much as to take turns talking and we do all this vocalization talking in our own heads which makes it very difficult to hear the other person. We have a hard time shutting down our minds and listening to our own thoughts to listen to somebody else's. It's a skill and it's not our fault. We were never trained to do this. You know my martial arts instructor trained me how to do this but I don't know of anybody else that was really trained how to do this. So we have a lot of challenges in this area and the solution is to listen intensely and let your own thoughts go into the story and visualize what the person is telling you. Listen to all the nuances. Remember the words they're saying, the tone of the body language, listen to the values, and the essence of the message. Become a very good listener.

The only way you're going to become a great communicator. How can you respond back when you don't even know what they said? And how can you come up with the right message when you don't know what they said? You can't be a great listener. You'll be a great communicator. I'll see you in the next chapter. And we got an awesome series of tips to kind of wrap up this chapter for you. And I'll see you there. Take care.

Still MORE Great Tips! Part 1

Hey everybody, welcome back to this chapter we're just going to do some great tips to kind of wrap up this Book for the last couple of chapters. Just some fun tips, some great tips, some things that really push ahead and give you the communication style that you always wanted. So let's jump right in. Now the first one is a powerful one to show appreciation for other people's ideas, experiences and feelings. Why? Because this is literally who they are. The likability factor we talked about this earlier is huge if we hang out with people we know like and trust we listen to and are influenced by people we know like and trust we listen to people who we know like and trust like and trust are the biggest things. And which comes first. You think she trusts you, like you probably are going to get far enough in a communication unless you've known somebody for a long time that they're going to trust you.

But likability can happen almost instantly and they can feel like they know you almost instantly. So you get two out of three pretty quick and maybe a little bit of trust but that may be for different chapters. So here's how you gain a huge amount of likability. People are in love with their ideas. Right, wrong or indifferent you're probably never going to change your ideas and they're just waiting. They are starved for people to show appreciation for their ideas. They also think their experiences are wildly valuable even though they're probably fairly typical experiences. They wouldn't be describing them to you if they didn't have a huge significance to them. Therefore it should have the same level of significance to you. It's simple appreciation. People love it.

And how about if somebody told you about their feelings and you didn't appreciate it. How would they feel completely unappreciated if not humiliated and embarrassed. So you always have to show appreciation for their feelings and you also have this if you want to show appreciation for who they are don't just reflect on oh that must have been a horrible experience. Talk to them about how much strength they must have had and how much character they must have had. Talk about who they are in this experience.

That must have made you so much stronger. You know I wish I had those kinds of strengths. I don't wish that experience on anybody but I wish for that strength that showing appreciation of who they are and that's the highest level of appreciation because you can like somebody has ideas you can like their clothes their shoes their experiences you can you know give homage to their feelings but what they really want you to care about what they really want you to like what they really want to appreciate is what them who they are. Their very essence is great communication. Compliments compliments are interesting.

I read a study where people don't care if you're lying or not. Your star value with that person will still go up. They can know you're amazingly full of B.S. and they still like you better. This is how star people are for compliments so compliments are great for increasing likability and it makes people more open to what you have to say because they want to hear more. It's a big factor in likability which we said is huge. So we're more likely to listen to and be influenced by people we like. Now to get the best compliments what you want to do is you want to make sure that you're complimenting the person. I always give the example. Hey nice shoes.

Well did you compliment the person maybe in a backhanded kind of way. You really just complimented their shoes and they're not going to get excited that you like their shoes. They gave me a slight backhanded compliment in terms of they had to select those shoes they had to pick those shoes they had to search for those shoes. So it's a compliment to them in that way but it's very weak. Now if I say wow those shoes look great on you. Now I didn't compliment the shoes I complimented you. If I say nice dress I compliment the dress. If I said You look amazing in that dress I just complimented you not the dress. Which one do you think people would want you to compliment more? The dress. Wear them. They always want you to complement them. Same thing when you're out on the golf Book. Oh my god that was an amazing shot.

You complimented the shot. You say I can't believe you made that amazing shot. You're a fantastic golfer. I just complimented you and your golfing skills. That's a better compliment. I said the same thing. It was all about that last shot. But it's totally different to the person receiving it makes sense. Let's try to. Now this is a very important chapter because it's how to use conversations to build the rapport to build the relationship to get somebody to feel closer to you. And this is a great thing to use in your relationships very sincerely because your relationships will get stronger. They'll be kinder, more loving, more beneficial to you and to them a true win-win if ever there were a couple of conversation tips. Listen to and tell stories people love. I'll have an actual little chapter on this and why stories are so important but very important that you listen to the stories because stories are adventures that people have.

It's again something that is important to them. It's also important to tell stories because now you're sharing a little bit of yourself with the other person. Hopefully it is a little bit of a moral to the story or chapter or a back end I call it you know kind of a take away something that they can learn from the story both about you and maybe about life as well. I'm a teacher so I tend to go that way but that's ok. Giving praise. Very similar to giving compliments. People are constantly doing things that are praiseworthy but we don't give them the praise. It's almost like we're being cheap with it. Like if we get so many praises if we give mouth they will run out. No you don't run out of praise that you can give to people you don't want to overdo it you don't want to over ingratiate. But when you notice somebody doing something nice, a boy that was really nice to you. Very simple but very powerful.

Share small secrets, members we said we want to communicate well with and we connect with people that we know, like and trust. And we said that knowing a sense that I know who you are and likability. We said those two come pretty easy. The hardest one was trust. Here's a way to start building trust. And you do it in a scale and proportionate way of sharing small secrets. You want to be talking about sexual positions that you like on the first date you know or with someone you don't know but you might share a small secret. I dress my dog up for Halloween. Kind of dumb and embarrassing but I did it. Ok that one you can share. OK. So you look for small secrets that you can share that give people a sense that you're trusting them a little bit then they'll trust you a little bit and they will share a little bit more with you. The more you share with them the more they share with you. This reciprocity goes and this creates trust. Great great way to do it.

Sharing goals are the things that are most important to you. If you share your goals with them, guess what they're probably going to reciprocate and are going to start talking about their goals. And certainly after you've talked about your goals you can give him the opportunity to talk a little about their goals, their goals or the major things they want in life. How valuable is that to knowing in a conversation if you're trying to be influential with somebody. And isn't this sharing because these things are very important when you're sharing something that's very important with somebody that creates trust. That second thing that's hard to get is to share small bits of personal information. So it might not necessarily be a secret but you can share little things.

Hey here's what I do for a job. Here's what I used to do when I was growing up. Here's one fun thing I used to like to do. Here's a little bit of information about one of my siblings or you know I have three dogs. You know whatever little bit of personal information is things you like to do like to go fishing, golf camping, whatever it is. Share a little bit of that again as people know personal details. They feel like you're sharing things instead of hiding things. Hiding things creates concern and distrust sharing things and giving little tidbits of personal information creates knowing and therefore trust and comfort demonstrate liking. Who do you like the most? The people who demonstrate that they like you hug you and they kiss.

They slap you on the back, they tell you jokes, they get a big smile on their face when they see you know they just love you to death. They demonstrate liking over and over and over and over and over again. So you need to demonstrate some liking when they tell you stories say boy I really like that you know. I like that you do this. You can use the word like you know but you can demonstrate liking in a lot of different ways just by smiling and agreeing I can demonstrate somebody I like by picking up the check. There's a lot of ways to demonstrate liking but make sure you're doing it. We always forget this in communication. I try never to forget it. Note similarities when we said we know we connect with people that we know, like and trust. Here's what we typically know like and trust people and have the good taste to be just like us. Salesmen used to use this as a technique I'm sure they still do.

They would look around your office or your house. They would see something that matched up with something that was in their life and they would note it all if you like golf.

I like all of you like dogs I like dogs you like cats I like cats. Boom boom boom boom boom. Hopefully it was very sincere. But people are always telling you things and you're going to have at least a 20 to 30 percent overlap just noted. Oh he likes that. I really liked that too when I was a kid I started doing blah blah blah blah and you know that's how I got into that book. Let them tell their story back about how they got into it. Note the similarities. The more you are like them the more they're going to like you. The last one uses humor.

Nobody defends against humor. Humor can tell little stories. Humor helps people have a good time. Why are people conversing anyways for no godly reason unless they're forced to be stuck in a room with you. This is like a mandatory court order. You want people to have a good time. People have a good time when you make them feel good about themselves and when you make them happy. So my goal when I'm with anybody is to make them have a good time. So listening to them makes them happy, complimenting them makes them happy. Having that human connectedness with them makes them happy and telling jokes makes them happy you know. Or even enjoying their jokes. Maybe they're the funny ones and you're the less funny ones. Enjoy their sense of humor and you will have a good time. If you're having a good time we like to match the people that we're with.

If you're smiling more they'll smile more laugh more they'll laugh more you are a little more trusting they'll be a little more trusting here a little bit more energetic. There'll be a little more energy. So in the LP Neuro-Linguistic program we call this matching and mirroring. You can match to the other person but you can also get the other person to match you. You can stick things up a notch and make them a little happier. Make them a little more energetic. They will love you for that. We never dislike people that we have a good time with. You know we're craving people to come into our lives and make us feel better without us having to do anything. That's a gift. So use humor whenever you can. And nobody defends against humor. As long as it's not too sarcastic I leave you that thought and I'll see you in the next chapter.

Still MORE Great Tips! Part 2

Hey everybody, welcome back. Now here's another great communication tip. Be positive. Why is this so important? The challenge is that if you talk about negative things people will get excited. They'll even join in the Go back and forth about the negativity and you'll think you're having a great conversation. But what's happening is and we learn this from neuro linguistic programming. An LP is that people will make neuro associations. It means one two things happen together they get linked up they get connected in our mind as being the same. So in this case you're being negative and they're looking at your face. They're being negative and they're looking at your face. There's negativity happening and they're looking at your face pretty soon.

Every time they look at your face they feel negative. It's not a good association. You want the opposite. Every time they see you you want them to feel positive just when you walk in the room. You want positive neuro associations not negative neuro associations. Remember people are always linking things up don't get linked to the negativity Don't be the bearer of bad news. Always be the bearer of good news. And remember we're trying to connect with somebody and have them like you to have likability. You're supposed to make the conversation more engaging, more fun, more empowering for them. There's very few ways to do that through negativity. So if he quit if he can't talk about something positive, skip the negative drive on and once again.

There's always something positive. Now here's the other key reason why you only want to have positive conversations. This is a great old therapy quote. It says very few people remember what you said but they always remember how you made them feel. So the major takeaway when they leave you is how you make them feel. Because literally we communicate with emotional messages. Remember those emotional messages. You want these to be positive abortion's always make people feel good about themselves, about their lives, about who they are and they will absolutely love you. So I always try to leave people with a good experience and on a good high note now tell stories. I tell stories because stories are very very powerful.

When we're little kids we learn from stories our dads tell us stories our moms tell us stories. We're literally designed to learn from and listen to stories. Stories are powerful because they get us to picture things. We have an emotional response to them. We get into the story. Stories make it easier to remember certain points because we've had a full body of experience. We pictured it. We felt that we've associated maybe with a character in the story. We are literally hardwired to learn from stories. So Stories are a great way to engage people, keep attention open and their minds make a point. It's an excellent communication strategy. Matter of fact, that's what most professional speakers do. They tell a story, tell a story, tell a story, make a point, link to another story, tell a story, tell the story, tell the story, and make a point.

Linked to another story tell the story tell the story tell a story make a point. Bull by time you're done. In about 45 minutes they've told four or five different 10 to 15 minute stories. The audience is absolutely engaged. They remember the three four or five points that were told to them and off they go and they say wow that was a brilliant speaker. Well he didn't do a lot of educating but these brilliant speakers know you can probably walk away with only one two or three messages anyways so you might as well spend that time instead of giving people 50 messages give him you know three or four because that's the most they're ever going to walk away with anyways and make those very engaging and lock them in by telling a story they know that's what holds the attention.

They know that's what creates retention and it's a great communication technique. So let's go over the list of why stories are great. First one is when we talked about this a couple of times that they do hold attention they are fantastic at holding attention like nothing else. Literally people don't defend against stories. So it's a way to get inside someone's mind without the normal objections and shields and biases and filters and everything else. That's a wonderful reason why stories are great. Retention: if you give out a dry cold fact it's very hard for people to remember. Human retention rates are about 4 percent. If you tell a story and they engage in the story then retention rates can be really high.

You know maybe half the audience or three quarters of the audience will remember the story and sometimes they'll remember the story for life. It has a very high retention rate. Not only you know a day later or 30 days later but years later they evoke emotion and emotion Locsin learning. Think about people who are traumatized and literally can't get rid of their thoughts. There was so much emotion at the time that it's with them for life. It haunts me every day. So emotion is huge. Emotion is great for locking and learning. Why do you remember your first kiss on your wedding day when your first child is born? You know a car accident because when anything is emotionally intense your body actually releases a chemical called Vasos Presa and it locks in memories. It's the hormone inside your body that decodes your memories. So even at low levels outside of scale how much Vasos presses it gets released.

So Stories are a nice low level way to release Vai's oppressiveness and lock in memories and lock in the learning people of stories because they're interesting cold dry facts that are boring and are difficult to remember. Remember we're hardwired to learn from stories. Therefore they're more interesting to us. They're more engaging and they lock in the memories better. And finally and this is the biggest reason they helped to drive home points. You know they really contain good solid chapters that people can learn from. And it's a way to give people an emotional reason why a motive which we said is the root word of motivation for why they should do something. So stories more than facts tend to get people to actually get up and take action.

And that's what we want when we're communicating with people we don't want to communicate just to communicate and share information. You could do that with a letter or hand them a book when we're communicating. We want them to take some kind of action. Stories are the best for this that are your tips for today. And I'll see you in the next chapter.

Still MORE Great Tips! Part 3

Hey everybody, welcome back. Here's a few more tips to make your communication even more powerful. So the first one is to use quotes to add credibility quoting people that are more powerful than you to have more initials after their name that have more notability that are famous that are known to be highly intelligent. I love to use it. Einstein had a great quote that said Genius is the ability to reduce the complicated to the simple. The reason you're using quotes is to borrow intelligence. The credibility of somebody else like Einstein lets the smartest guy in the whole world be right but pretty smart.

So people are going to listen to Einstein because they figure they're not smarter than Einstein so they may not believe something that you say but they certainly will believe something that Albert Einstein says. Quotes can be a great way to add credibility in quotes and are a great way to condense knowledge. An entire large concept into like a single sentence or two like this is a large concept. Genius is the ability to reduce the complicated to the simple. So what you're doing is you're taking something complex and you're making it easier to understand. So this is a concept for simplifying say your business or if you're Speaker you should be able to reduce things down to the third grade level so that everybody can understand it and you're actually seen as a bad speaker.

If you can't do that you're stuck up your snobbish you're losing people the whole way. So great communication has to do with quotes and it also has to do with reducing the complicated to the simple. So two great tips and one. Let's move on to the next one. People understand this I think intuitively but they often forget about it. Is that the way that we dress? Is actually a form of communication. Your first impression happens within the first seven seconds. People have decided about 90 percent of what they're going to decide about you in the first seven seconds. So Visual Communication is actually huge. It's not an afterthought. It's something that you really need to focus on. Always give a good first impression. They say you don't get a second chance to make a first impression. That's true.

I suppose you can go back and clean it up afterwards but it's really difficult. You know that's really paddling uphill. So you always want to make a great first impression. Best way to do it. Dress your best, look your best and act your best. Does that mean groom properly with no dirt under the nails? I always take a shower before you leave the house. Make sure you smell good so you don't smell too good and smelly from across the room if you're a woman. And I'm further than one foot away. I shouldn't be able to smell you coming into the room. So you also want to make sure that you get the right impression.

So match the environment if you should be wearing a suit. Make sure you're wearing a suit. You should be wearing shorts make sure you're wearing shorts. So always match the environment and always dress about one tier above everybody else. You know one tier above at least what the median is. So you look like you're in a slightly upper tier. You never wish you were one tear down that will leave the opposite impression. Another crucial one. I love this picture here, don't you? Be sure to avoid any judgmental statements or words. What judgemental statements or words. Well I'm glad you asked a lot of times.

Good or bad, right or wrong can be very judgmental. Sometimes they're not. These aren't words you always have to avoid but sometimes you want to avoid them if they're coming off as judgmental. So look out for words like good or bad right or wrong. Always always is. It's one of those odd words that makes such a definitive statement. There's no wiggle room in that. This always happens most of the time when you always say you're wrong. Should should means you should have done this. You didn't do it and therefore your bad can't become a word that makes things and possibly can't do this you can't do that. It puts value judgments on people as well.

Evil is another powerful one. There's more words like this. Here's some straight up judgmental words. Stupid dumb. You must do this, you must do that. Calling somebody you know a geek or a jock is no good. Never you better or. That's ridiculous. These are judgmental statements or words would be very very cautious with ease. They can really hurt you in the long term. Just be very cautious around them. So those are your tips for today and I'll see you in the next chapter.

Conclusion

Hey everybody, welcome back. I can't believe we're at the end of the chapter. Here's your final tips. Congratulations you made it all the way through the Book. You're in the top 10 percent of the top 10 percent which puts you in the top 1 percent. You do it absolutely amazing. So let's jump right in and get you these final tips. Here's a great one. Remember this and write it down. Actions speak louder than words. There's an old quote that says who you are speaks so loudly I can't hear what you're saying. That's the same as saying Your actions speak so loudly I can't hear what you're saying. People when they have to choose between something that you say and something that you do for sincerity they're going to believe what you do.

We used to teach this to family members of clients who are addicted. We would say don't listen to a thing they say and read everything they do. They say they're going to a meeting. You say that's nice but you don't believe them. They're coming back from a meeting and they're describing the meeting to you and telling you about what happened in the meeting. That's real. Give him credit for that. They say they're going to call a sponsor. You say that's nice. They get off the phone with the sponsor. That's real. Same with your kids. They say you're going to clean their room. You say that's nice. They finish cleaning their room. That's what you believe. Actions always speak louder than words. Actions are the best form of communication.

If you say you're going you're in a conversation with somebody and you're going to say you're going to help them take an immediate action get a phone number for them make a note to yourself to make something happen the next day to make the phone call to fill out a piece of paperwork to do something something something that's an actual action step. You say you're going to connect them with somebody, give them their phone number or make a quick call and say hey this is i want to leave a quick voicemail and to have my friend Johnny call you tomorrow. Please take his call. He's a great guy and I'll talk to you soon, my friend. Goodbye Bill. You took action to tell your friend. I'm going to connect you with my buddy here. That's one thing you take that action in front of him.

So now you've got absolute confidence that these things are going to happen. Powerful communication technique Here's that quote again who speaks so loudly I can't hear what you're saying. How will you always be seen in the right light? Act the way you want to be seen, speak the way you want to be seen. Do the things that show the way you want to be seen. It's called congruency. Make sure that everything you're doing in your communication, your facial expressions, your words, your actions, your follow-ups, all put you on the side of the angels as we look at this picture here and our congruency.

You don't want to say one thing, do another that will shatter the communication, shatter the trust, shatter the relationship, everything should match up. Now quick shameless plug here. I've got some great chapters that will add to this communication. Motivation is a great one. You can't do the slightest thing until you're motivated. So if you want to learn how to use communication to motivate yourself and others, the motivation one is absolutely fantastic is one of my best selling Books. If you want to make the motivation one and the communication want even more powerful. These all become synergistic together. Get the persuasion strategies one. I had a lot of fun doing this one. It's all about specific tools, strategies and techniques to help yourself be more persuasive to get people to take a certain action.

You can use these techniques on yourself and you can use them on other people. I always work it both ways so you get double the benefit from all my chapters and that you can be massively successful. My chapter is designed so that you have an unfair advantage. So I leave you with this. What is the world's greatest communication tool? Think about it. What do you think it is? It's to be a great friend. If you simply look at every communication you have as if you're having it with your best friend you'll always come across as somebody they know, like and trust and that knows likes and trusts them.

That is literally the ultimate in good communication. So all the way through your communication. I want you to be thinking of the person across the table from you as your best friend. If you do that you'll do absolutely amazing and you will be a master communicator. So if you have any questions you purchase this Book. I want to help you out. I want to give you additional background information. Answer any questions you have. Did I pose for this picture is not a legitimate question but any other questions. Go ahead and use the message system within the platform that you purchased.

I usually check those about once a day or once every other day so you'll be able to communicate with me. I will get back to you as quickly as I can. If you have a second or third question you can get as many as you want. Go ahead and send them to me. We love to hear from you. My name is Professor . There's my good buddy JJ here with me, my corporate mascot and I hope to see you in my next chapter. Get out there and be a master communicator.

Don't miss out!

Visit the website below and you can sign up to receive emails whenever Gaurav Sanjiv Kalangan publishes a new book. There's no charge and no obligation.

https://books2read.com/r/B-A-EPFBB-ISPZC

Also by Gaurav Sanjiv Kalangan

Learn Options Strategies Options Basics & Greeks For Stock Trading By Technical Analysis
Bitcoin, Altcoins & ICOs Learn the Basics of Digital Coins from Zero
Time Management This Is How I Work 300 Percent Faster
How To Build And Implement A Winning Pricing Strategy
Networking For Introverts: Gracefully Exiting A Conversation
Accounting 101: Learn Cost Accounting From A To Z
Growth Marketing: Strategy & Execution Bootcamp For Startups
Develop The Mental Strength Of A Warrior For Success In Life

www.ingramcontent.com/pod-product-compliance
Lightning Source LLC
Chambersburg PA
CBHW072213150726
48002CB00005B/1791